Detailed Specifications of The Brain Decoding Device.

Volume II

A Complete

Step-by-Step

Guide.

David Gomadza

First Global President of The World

Detailed Specifications of The Brain Decoding Device. Volume
II A Complete Step-by-Step Guide.

Copyright © 2023 David Gomadza

PAPERBACK ISBN: 9798862571875

This is volume II where I go deeper showing you all the possible uses and specifications of the brain decoding device.

Tomorrow's World Order
David Gomadza
I am the First Global President of the World.
00447719210295
info@twofuture.world
www.twofuture.world

Thoughts to Word or Audio [Brain Code]
Decoding the brain made easy. Breakthrough: we can communicate using thoughts.
Visit www.twofuture.world

Read the complete book series.
https://play.google.com/store/books/series?id=a4Mv GwAAABBFmM

Get and Install our Brain Code App
https://play.google.com/store/apps/details?id=com.ni otron.dgomadza.Brain_Code

Detailed Specifications of The Brain Decoding Device. Volume
II A Complete Step-by-Step Guide.

DEDICATION

Still to a better, more technologically advanced world.

Table of Contents

Detailed Specifications of The Brain Decoding Device. Volume II A Complete Step-by-Step Guide.

ACKNOWLEDGMENTS

Always thanks to Tomorrow's World Order.

CHAPTER ONE

You can test our brain decoder using the DIY gadgets listed below for less than $45.

Yes. A brain decoder for as little as a meal out. This is the future. You will all thank me later. This is what you will need, where to buy and how much this will cost you.

First this is the setting you must create at home as your workstation.

See volume 1 for more details.

The left side of the setting is what we are mainly concerned with here. Note it's the left side as you are sitting at a desk as below. This is the only way this will work without any further modifications. The right side is like a booster of the left side.

Don't worry about how complicated the diagram looks, see images inside. This is easy to setup once you have all the items. As a rule, get all the minimum parts needed. But there are a lot of other parts that can be added on top depending on what you are trying to achieve. That means we start as simple as possible. In the image below I replaced the actual brain decoding device that we will use at the end in the very advanced stages with a simple power-bank. If you want, you can recreate everything at the beginning, both the left and right sides. But at first, I will concentrate on the left side of this setting.

The Ultimate setting for the Brain
Decoding Device. It works tried and tested.

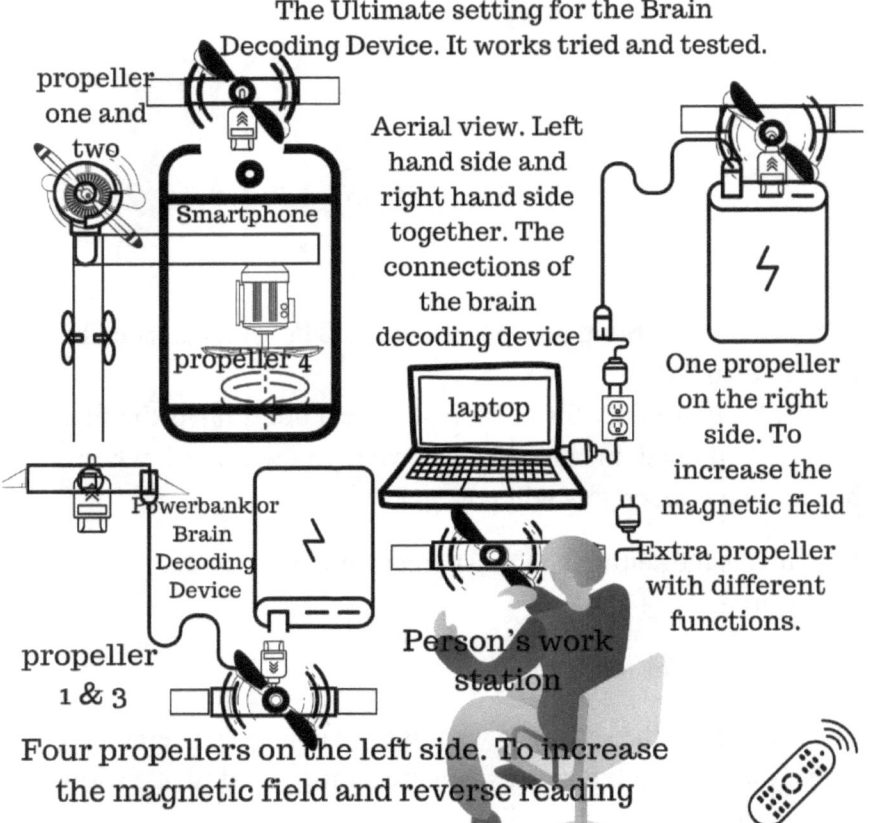

propeller
one and
two

Smartphone

propeller 4

Aerial view. Left
hand side and
right hand side
together. The
connections of
the brain
decoding device

laptop

Powerbank or
Brain
Decoding
Device

One propeller
on the right
side. To
increase the
magnetic field

Extra propeller
with different
functions.

Person's work
station

propeller
1 & 3

Four propellers on the left side. To increase
the magnetic field and reverse reading

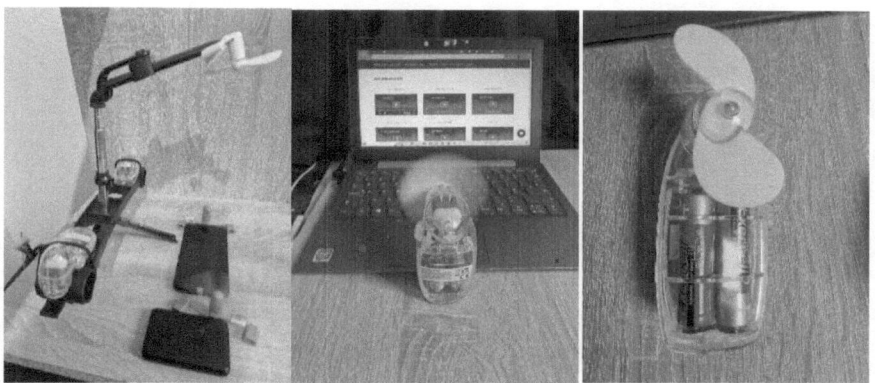

The Settings.

The Left side setting.

This is the critical side and care must be taken when setting up things on this side. This is what makes everything work. If it doesn't work for you then you must have made a mistake here.

The Center.

The Center that comprises of a laptop and the rotary propeller that is low but one that faces the laptop or computer screen. This must be at the center of the laptop screen and same level as the laptop.

The Right Side.

On the right side is the booster with one rotary propeller. You can use the same type of propeller but this one must be facing upwards like a helicopter blade as viewed from the top. The middle rotary propeller facing the laptop should be rotating facing the screen.

Any mistake cancels the flow of the electromagnetic waves so check carefully.

Task One.

This is what you will need to test and evaluate this brain decoder. Feel the power of the brain firsthand.

1. Your smartphone. That means everyone has one, which means that the cost is $0. But for advanced testing you will need an extra smartphone on which to use our brain code software to do deep brain decoding.
2. Oxy Cool 4" USB Mini fan product code SUM-3548 barcode 5056170335485 price $3 any Poundshop or online. Quantity x 1

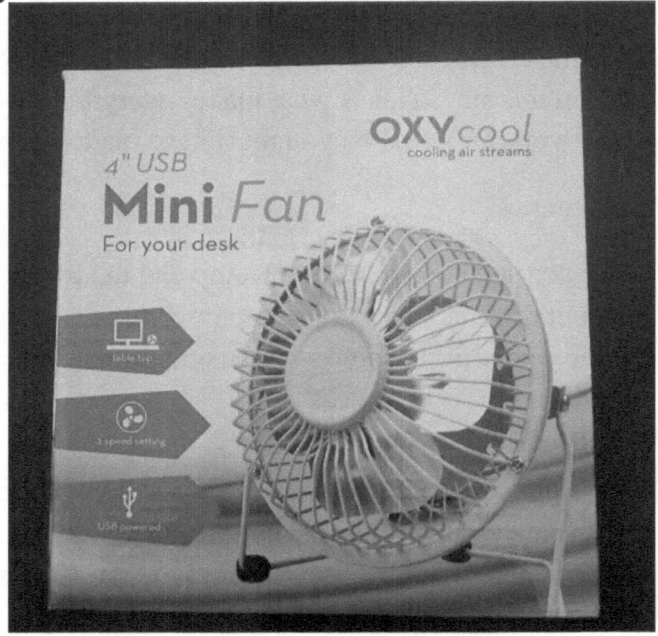

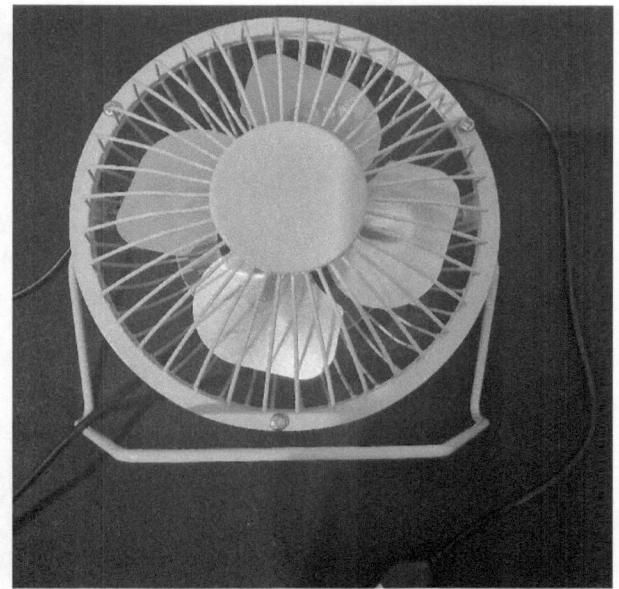

3. Oxy Cool Smartphone fan product code SUM-6721 barcode
    5056283867217 price $2
    Quantity 5 Total $10

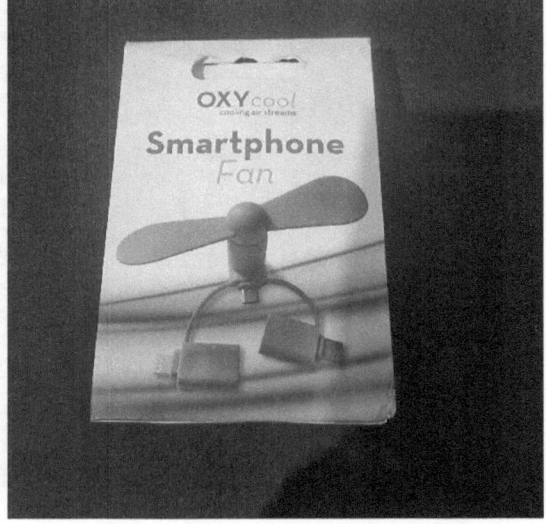

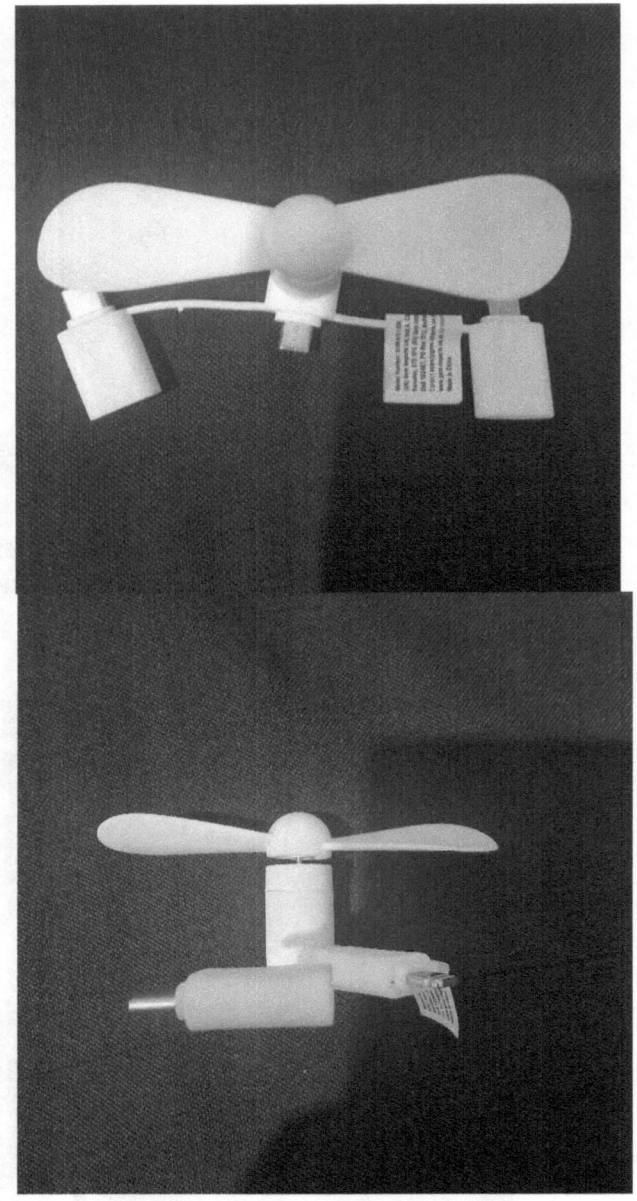

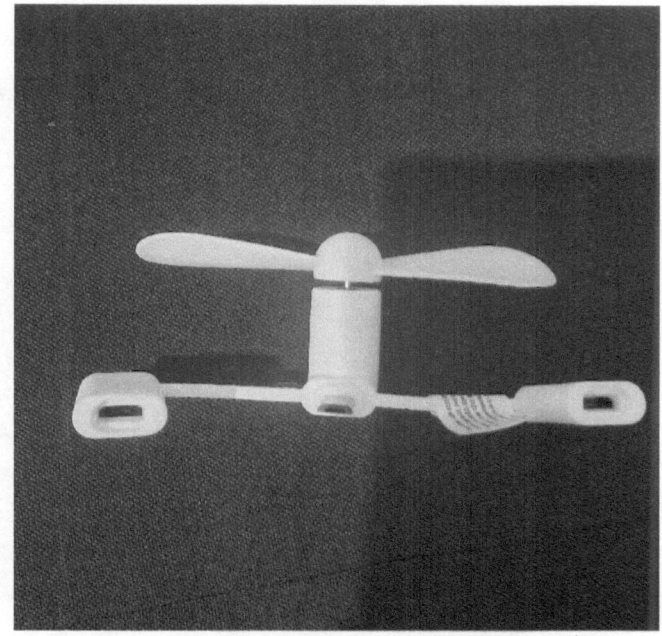

4. Any power bank or Juice Power bank x 2 each cost $10 Total $20.

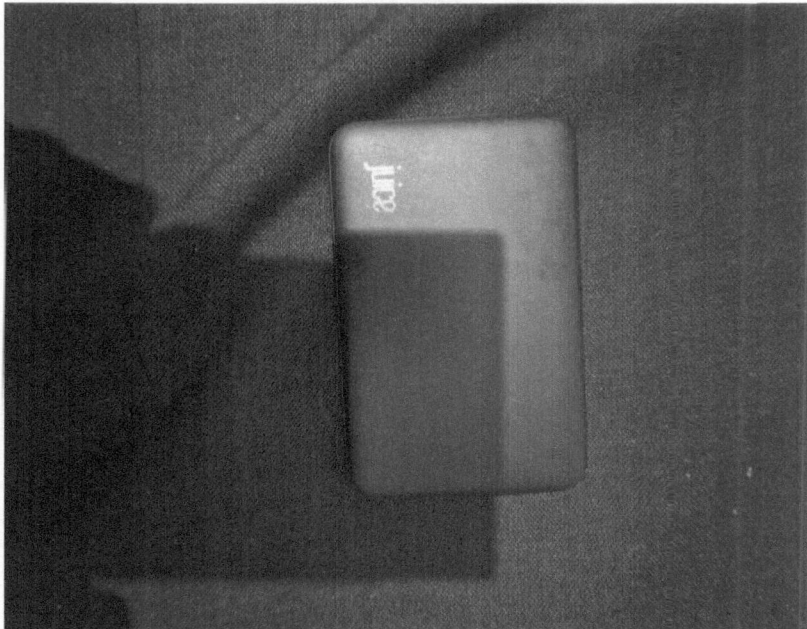

5. Viido wireless selfie-stick x 2

Cost $4 each
Total $8

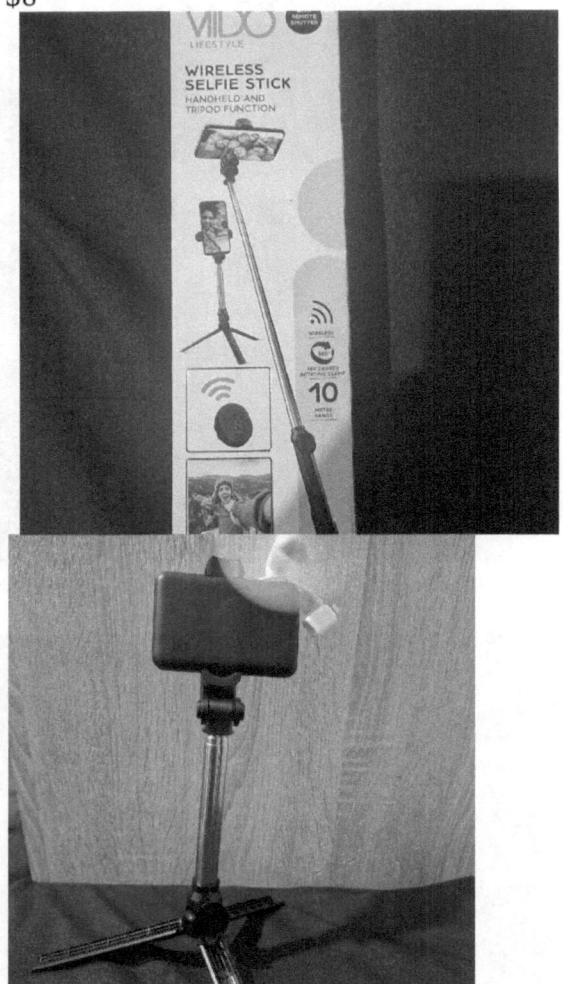

6. Wireless speaker WGO Bluetooth speaker $10 or any Bluetooth speaker.
7. A laptop or computer most people have already cost $0.
8. Universal gadget grip $2

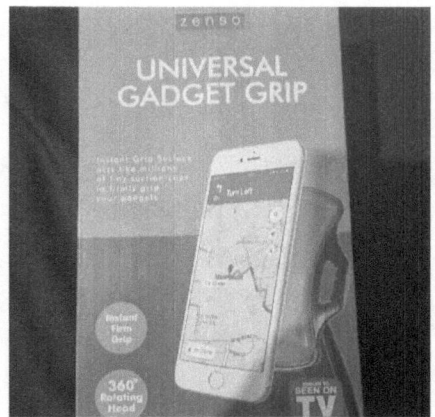

9. Video recorder software installed on your smartphone. Free from Google Play or Apple store Cost 0.

10. Voice recorder software installed on your smartphone. Free from Google Play Apps or Apple Store Cost $0.
https://play.google.com/store/apps/details?id=com.media.be strecorder.audiorecorder&hl=en_GB&gl=US

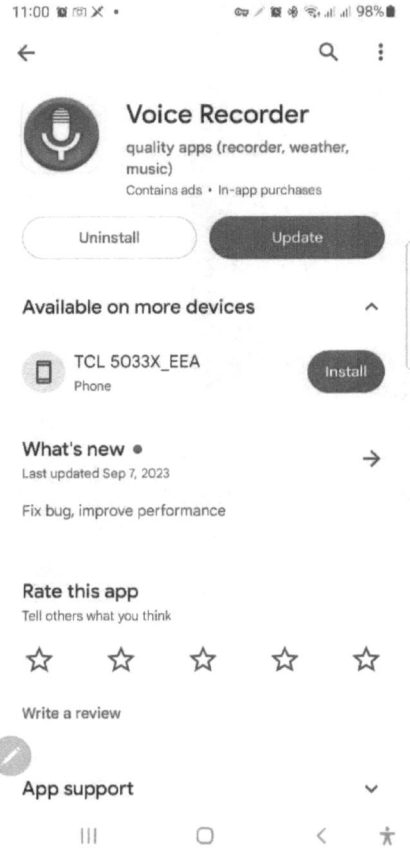

11. NCH software free trial. Wavepad.
    https://www.nch.com.au/wavepad/index.html

12. https://www.onlineconverter.com/increase-mp3-volume
    Access this website to convert and or amplify [increase the volume of an MP3].

13. Download the Brain Code App from Google Play.
    https://play.google.com/store/apps/details?id=com.niotron.d gomadza.Brain_Code&hl=en_GB&gl=US

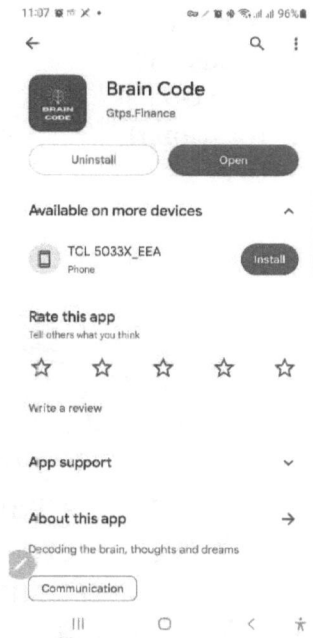

Stage One.

Emitting Your Thoughts Out of Your Body.

> The best thing about my Brain decoding device is that it does not need any operation on any part of your body. Yes, you heard me correctly. No medical procedure is needed. This is the way God intended humanity to be before he realized that the devil was a deceiving evil to trick Eve and condemn all humanity to sin. This has no side effects or anything adverse. It is the way nature intended. I explained in Volume I that God has a rotating earth on his right waistline. This is the only position in which he can receive all prayers from the earth as the earth rotates.
> Man was created in God's image meaning if we place man in place of God, we can recreate what does and happen to God and make it to also happen to people.

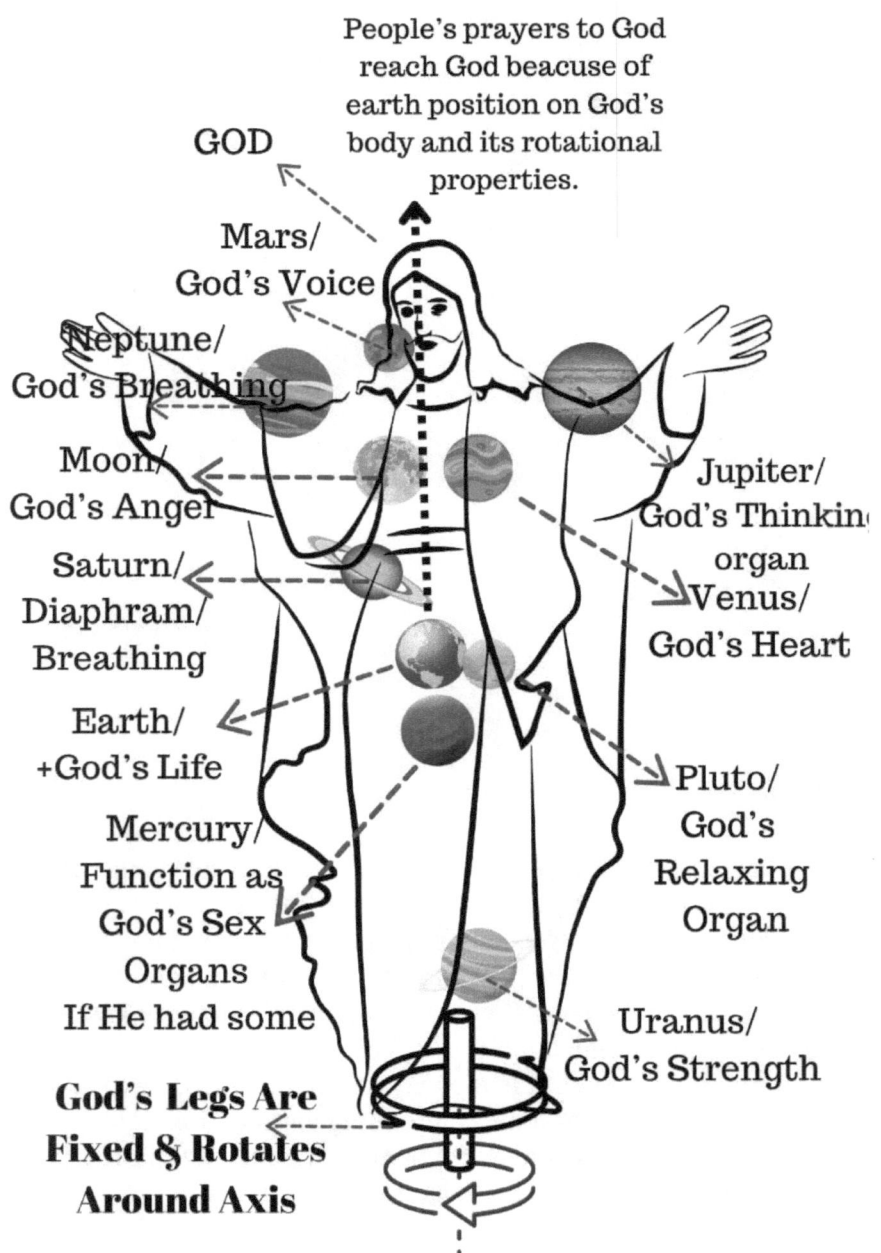

People's prayers to God reach God beacuse of earth position on God's body and its rotational properties.

GOD

Mars/ God's Voice

Neptune/ God's Breathing

Moon/ God's Angel

Jupiter/ God's Thinking organ

Saturn/ Diaphram/ Breathing

Venus/ God's Heart

Earth/ +God's Life

Pluto/ God's Relaxing Organ

Mercury/ Function as God's Sex Organs If He had some

Uranus/ God's Strength

God's Legs Are Fixed & Rotates Around Axis

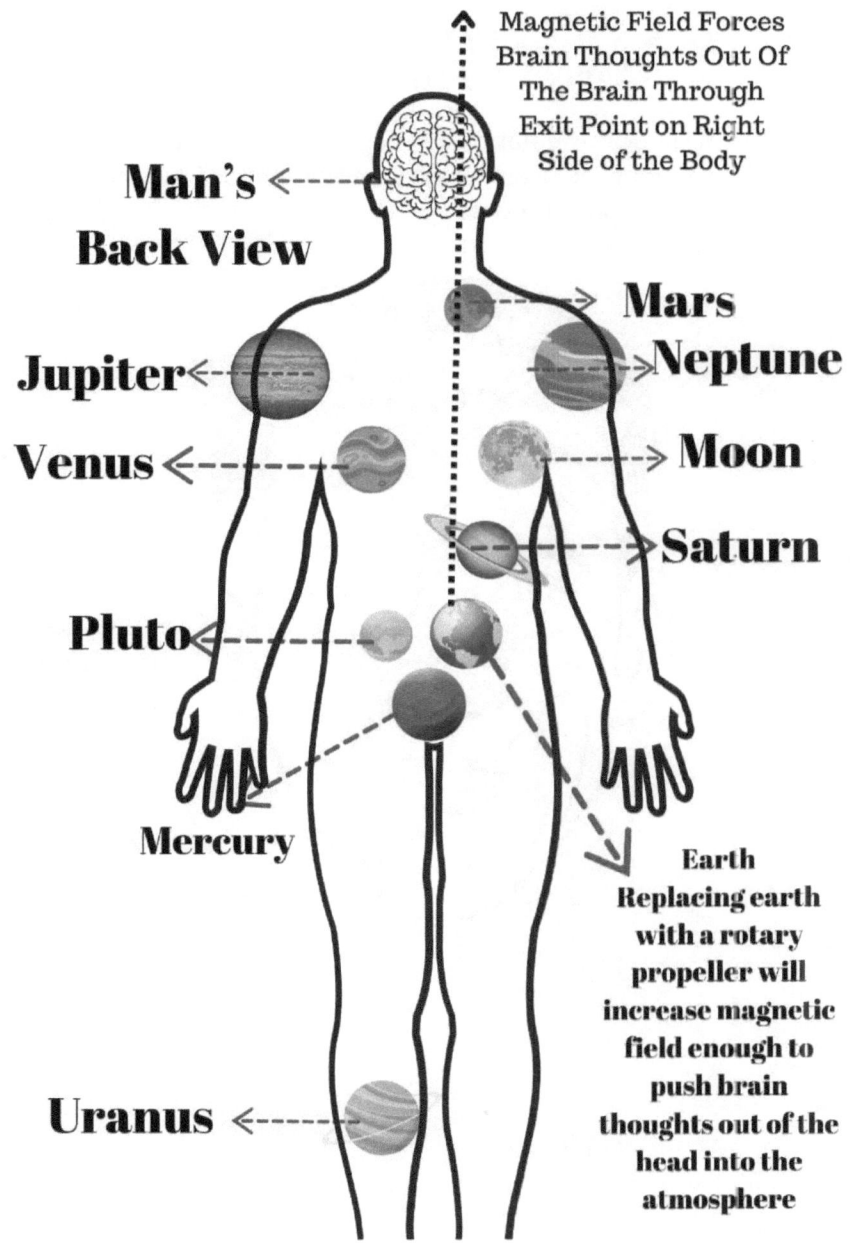

Magnetic Field Forces Brain Thoughts Out Of The Brain Through Exit Point on Right Side of the Body

Man's ← Back View

Mars

Neptune

Jupiter ←

Venus ←

Moon

Saturn

Pluto ←

Mercury

Uranus ←

Earth
Replacing earth with a rotary propeller will increase magnetic field enough to push brain thoughts out of the head into the atmosphere

Current Thinking Process

Brain thoughts generated in the brain are assembled on the
right side of the brain. These are not emitted out side of the
body but processed on the left side of the head.

Brain Thought Path

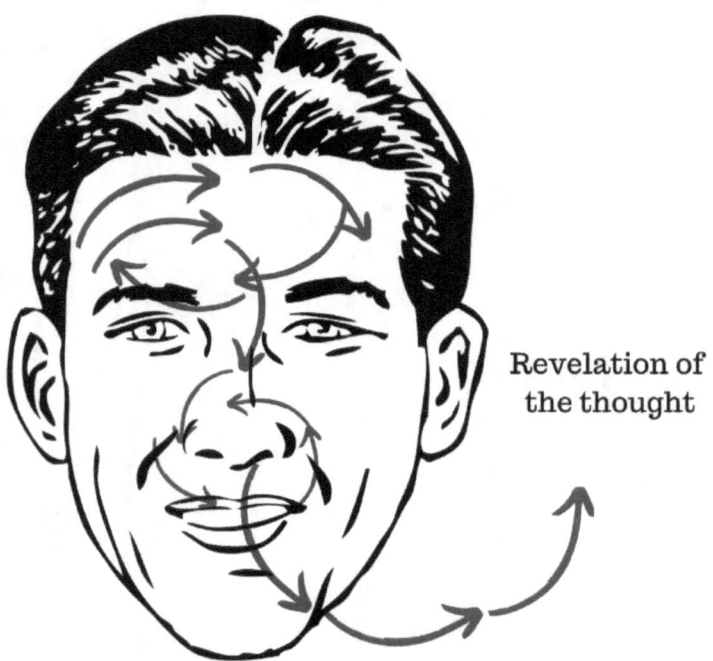

Revelation of
the thought

We want thoughts to be emitted outside of the head first.

Brain thoughts generated in the brain are assembled on the right side of the brain. Now we want to make these thoughts to be emitted outside of the body first and reentered into the brain through the entry point on the left side.

So how can we achieve this?

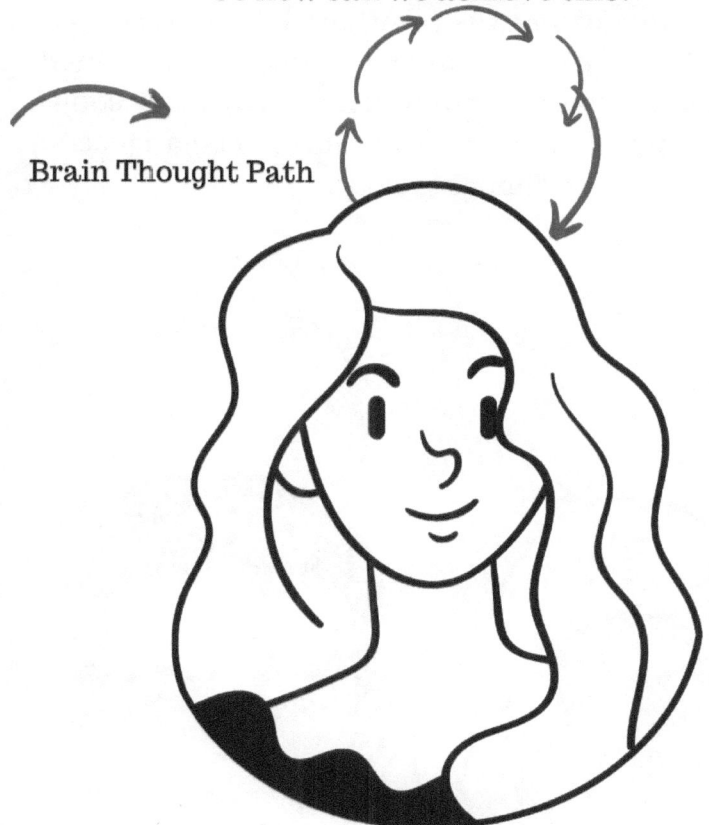

Brain Thought Path

But first why we want the brain thoughts to be emitted outside of the brain first?

To know what a person is thinking about. This is the only way to know because we can do a lot of stuff like for example capture and clone the thoughts before they are emitted back inside the brain to be processed.

As the brain absorbs the re-entered thoughts to be processed we can at the same time decode the cloned thoughts so that we know even before the person know himself or herself what he or she had just thought about.

Brain Thought Path

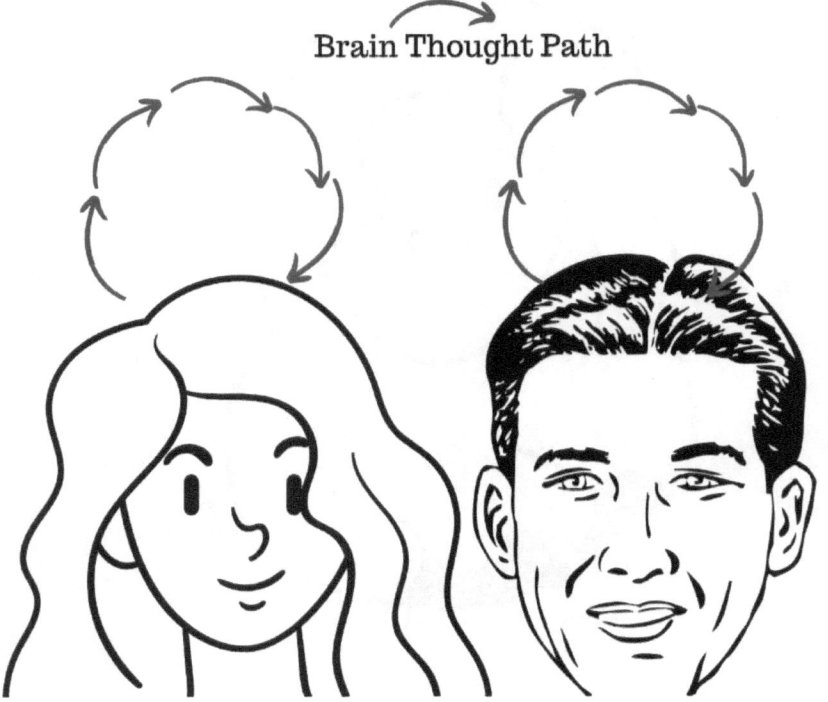

**Magnetic Field Forces Brain Thoughts Out
Of The Brain Through Exit Point on Right
Side of the Body**

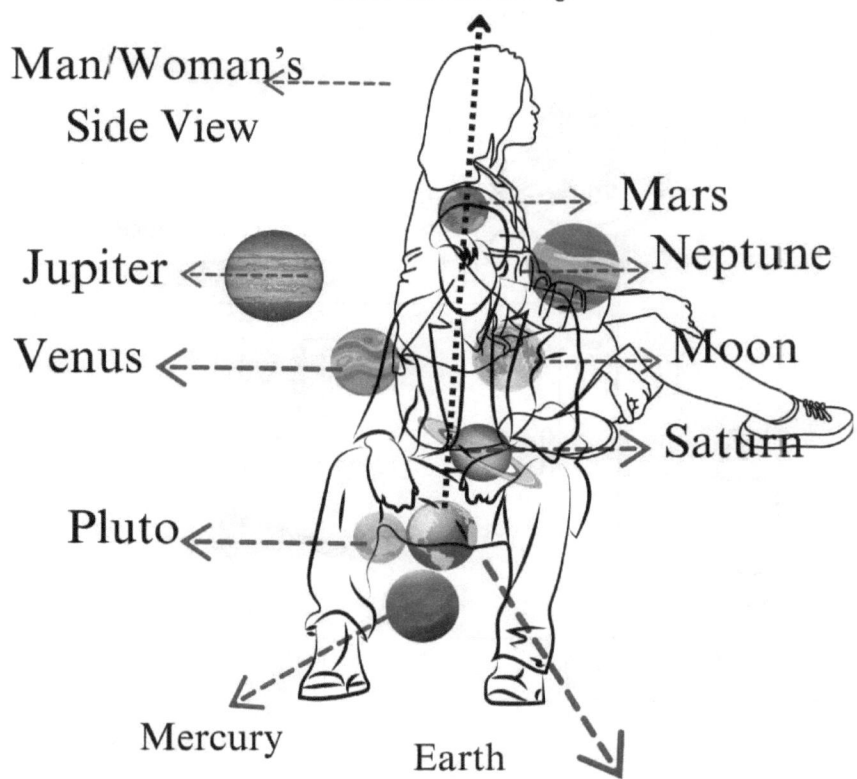

Man/Woman's
Side View

Jupiter

Venus

Mars

Neptune

Moon

Saturn

Pluto

Mercury

Earth

Replacing earth
with a rotary propeller will increase magnetic
field enough to push brain thoughts out of
the head into the atmosphere

Uranus

A rotating magnetic propeller acts as earth does
on God. Induce a strong magnetic field and push
peoples thoughts out of earth.

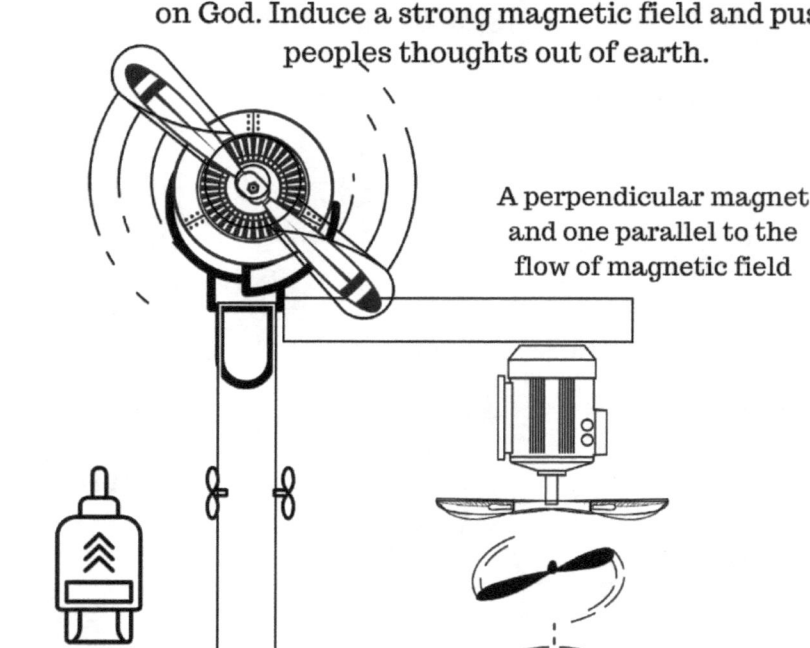

A perpendicular magnet
and one parallel to the
flow of magnetic field

Recall from volume one that electromagnetic propagation
creates a strong magnetic field that pushes forces out of the earth to
God in the case of God. Humans are created in God's image which
means if we replace the earth with the above rotary propellers, one
parallel to the direction of movement of the magnetic field and the
other at right angles or perpendicular this will push any
electromagnetic waves upwards.

Recall also that electromagnetic waves are the language of the brain. If we introduce the above settings of the two propellers in a human being this will push electromagnetic waves emitted from the limbic system of the brain out of the brain but instantly absorbed back into the body through the mouth if the mouth is open. The advantage here is that electromagnetic waves travel through solids, air, and even the vacuum of space.

We can therefore take advantage of this fact and reduce the processing time to compensate for the emission of brain thoughts outside of the body by making these thoughts be emitted straight into the body to the final processing system in the jaws through the mouth.

The position of everything as the solution.

The best position we can get is when a downward pointing magnet is under the buttocks of a sitting or squatting man as a right angle is created in line with the right-side center of the brain. So, this is the best position when a man is squatting. Recall what I said about God. People's thoughts are easily sent to God if they pray in a prostrate position with face down to the ground. That means that man's prayers are sent to the ground where they are then pushed to God by earth's rotational properties and a strong magnetic field.

The best setting for the propagation of the electromagnetic waves.

How do we push brain thoughts out of the human body?

Experiment 1 Practice This First.

What is needed for the experiment?
1. Two Oxy Cool Smartphone fans.
2. Oxy 4" USB Mini Fan
3. A chair.
4. A Viido wireless selfie stick.
5. A power-bank.
6. The universal gadget grips.

Do the following.
1. First place the Oxy 4" USB Mini Fan upside down
   underneath the right back side of the chair. Connect the
   Mini fan using the power on/off at the back. This can be
   connected to a laptop. This Mini fan has a mesh wire that
   will protect the rotary blades. Therefore, turn the fan upside

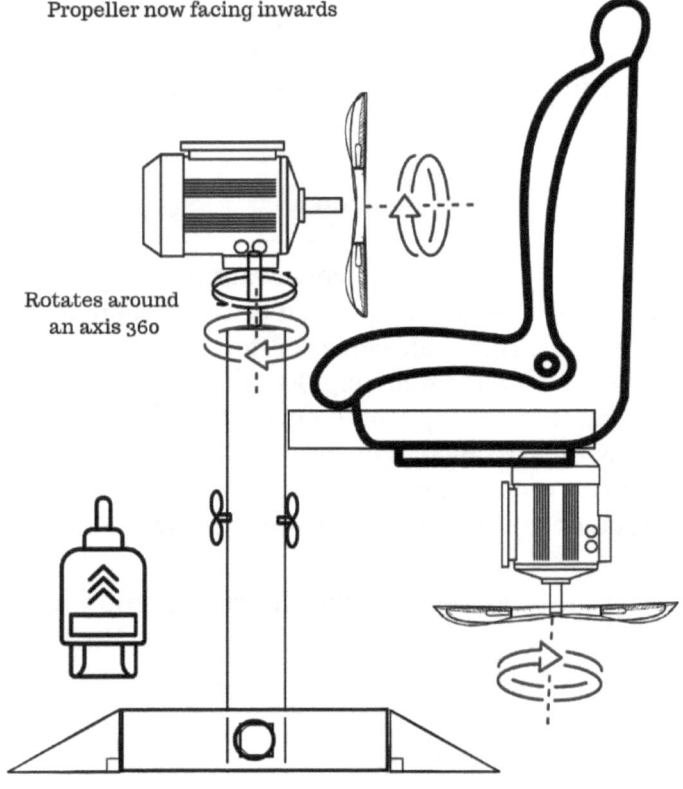

Propeller now facing inwards

Rotates around
an axis 360

down.

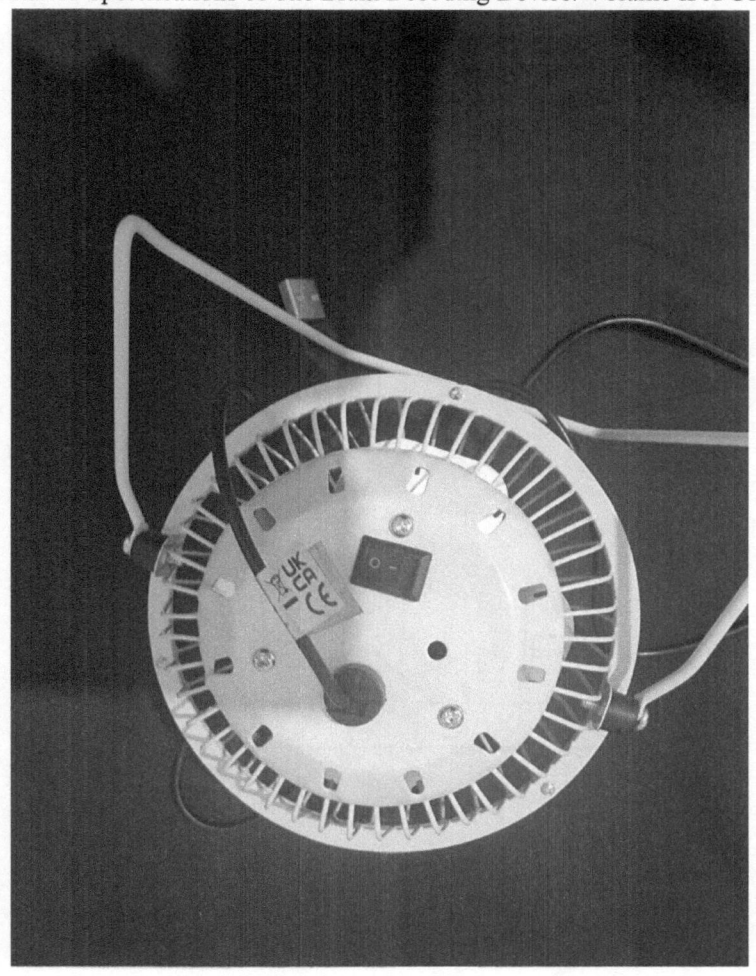

Invention 1 The Seat

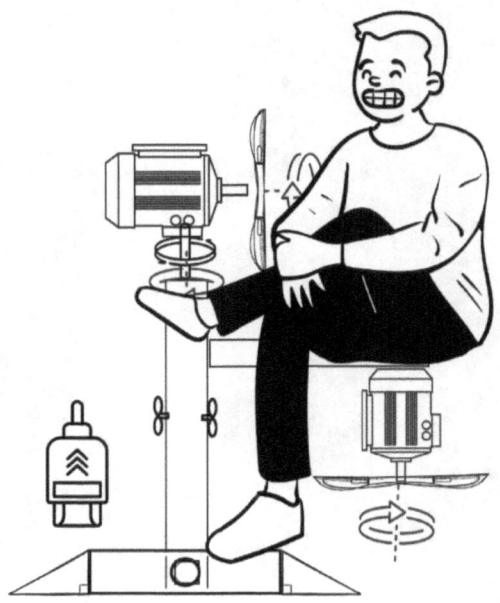

2. Connect the Viido wireless selfie stick. Place the Juice power-bank on it. Lastly, add one of the Oxy Cool Smartphone Fans. Careful placing this smartphone fan as there is no switch button. It starts to rotate the second it is connected to the power bank.

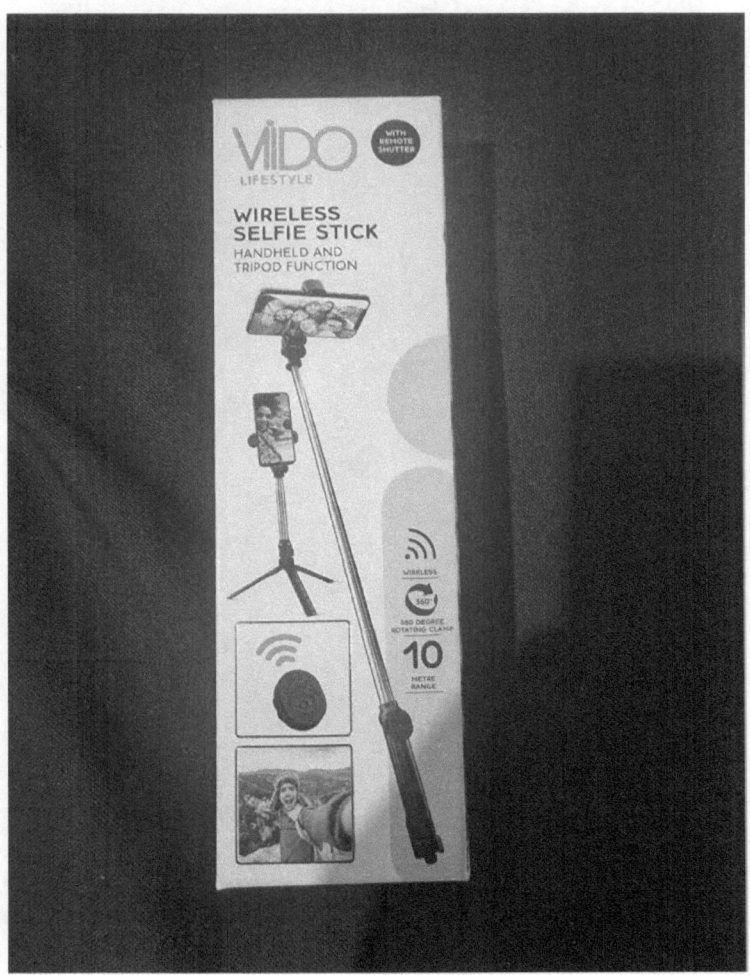

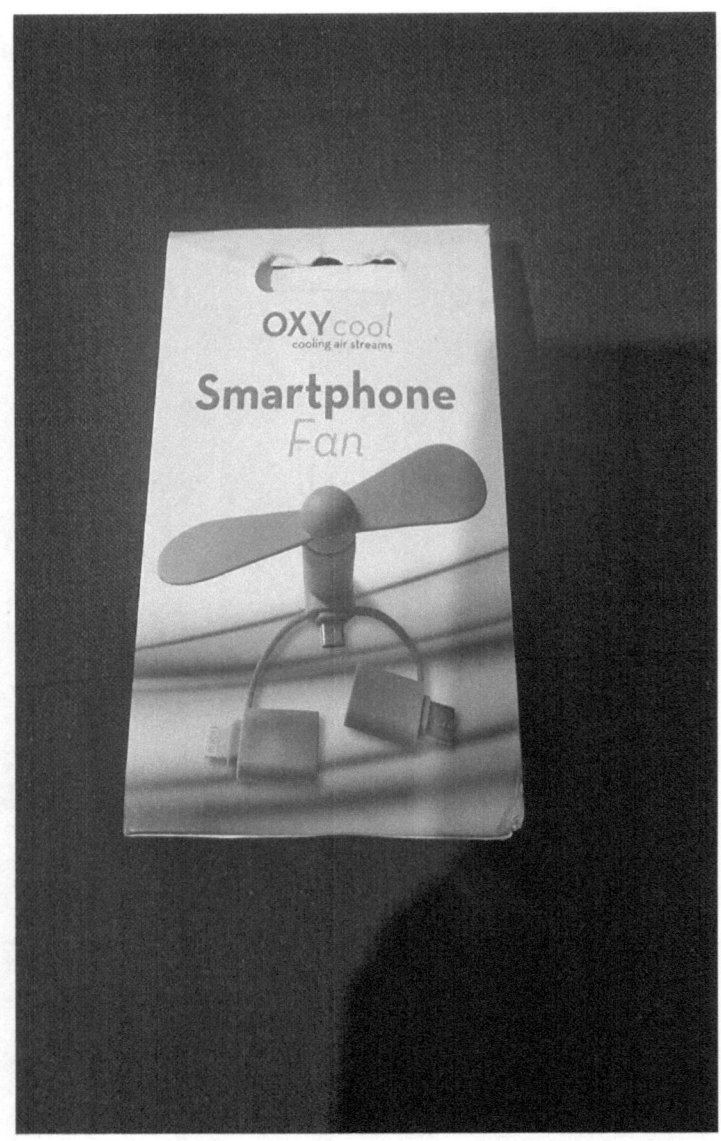

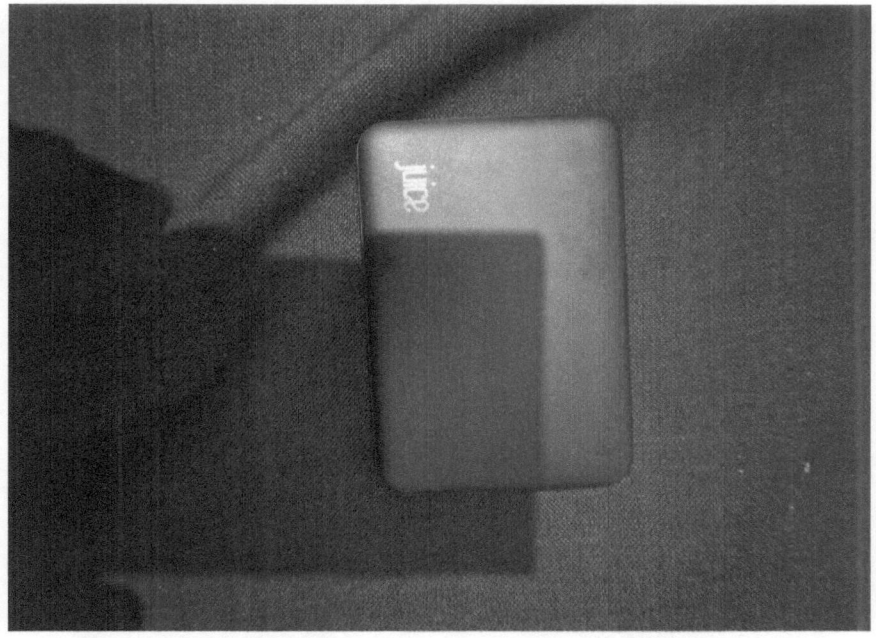

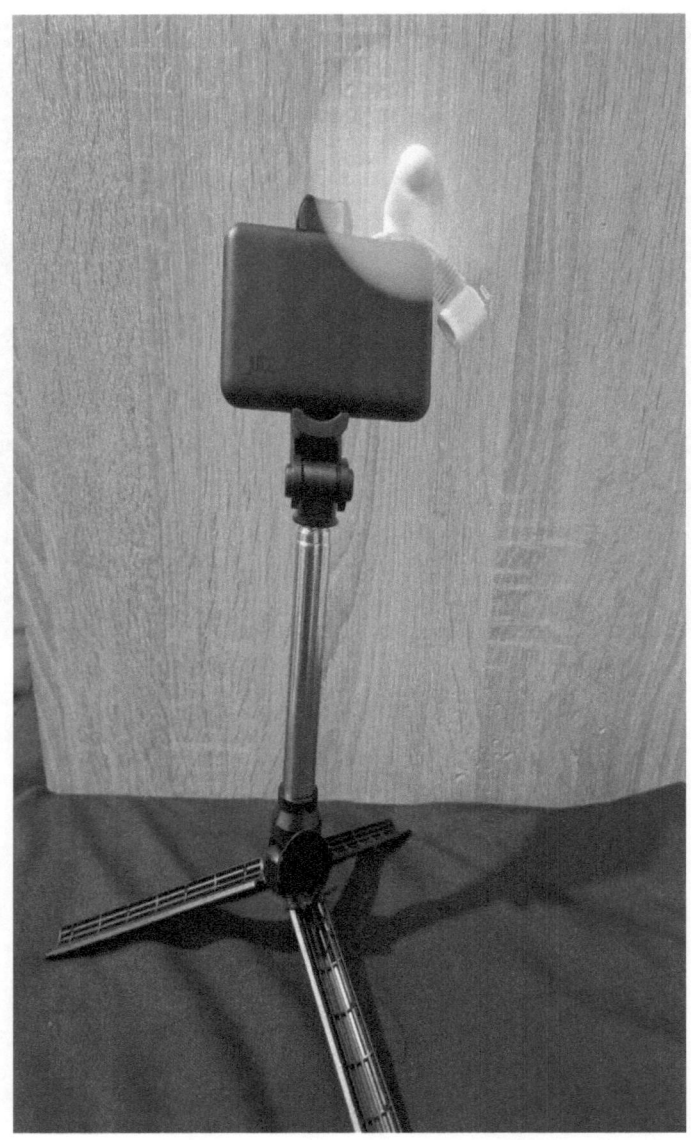

Invention 1 The Chair

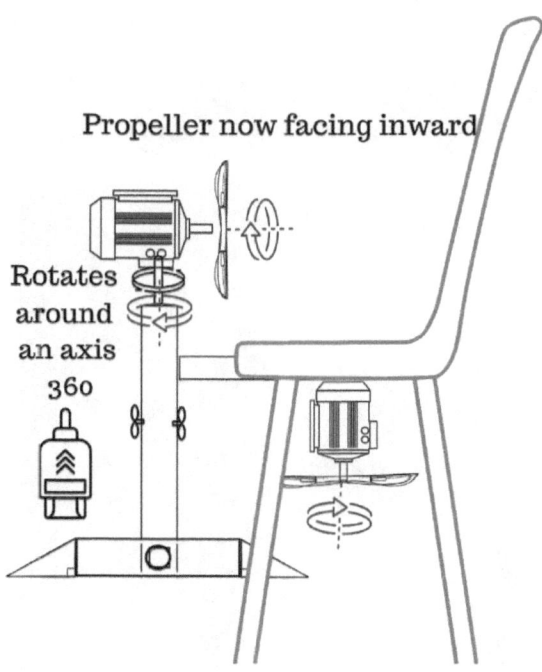

Propeller now facing inward

Rotates around an axis 360

The Oxy Mini fan is now under the chair on the right side back of the chair.

Now sit so that the right-side buttock part that sits and touches the chair seat is right at the bottom of the propeller. Place the Viido with the Juice Power-bank on it with an Oxy Smartphone fan or propeller connected. Take care when handling the propeller as it will start to rotate as it does not have an on and off button, you must be alert all the time. But remember it is made of rubber, even if it hits your hand, it will not cause any damage.

Place this selfie stick with the Juice power bank and the rotary Oxy smartphone fan in front of you on the working desk in front. Make sure the position is level with your mouth and keep a distance from you at least 20 cm away from you.

Make sure the rotary fan is away from you at least 20 cm from your body and remember it is not protected in that it does not have

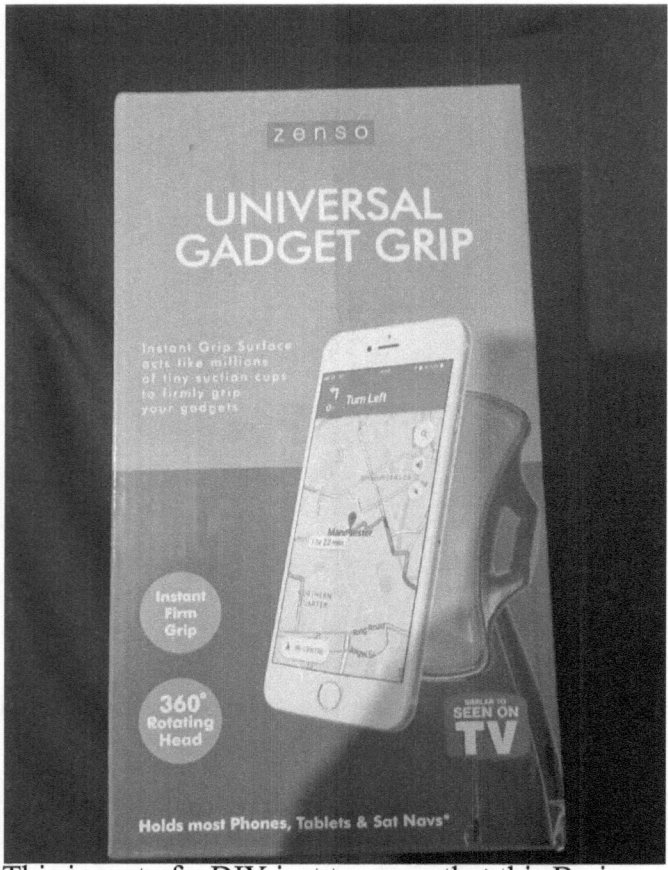

a cover. This is part of a DIY just to prove that this Brain Decoding Device works, and one does not need thousands of dollars to decode the brain.

See the below diagram for how this will appear.

Invention 1 The Chair

Propeller now facing inwards

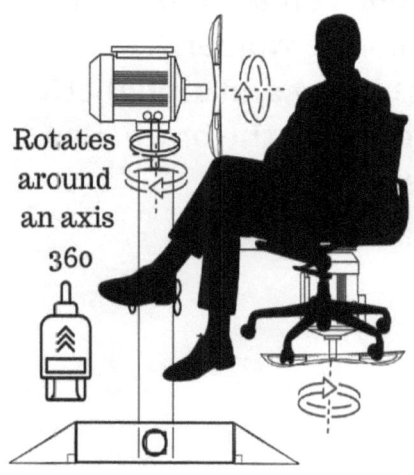

Rotates
around
an axis
360

Side view of the propagation of electromagnetic waves. The propeller has rotated and now facing inwards. The perpendicular propeller below it if turned on will enable the reverse reading and the backward mirror reading.
"Women are from Venus" will read "Venus from are women."
Read more about binary and alphabetic order assigning done by the brain. See earlier volumes.

Propeller now facing inwards

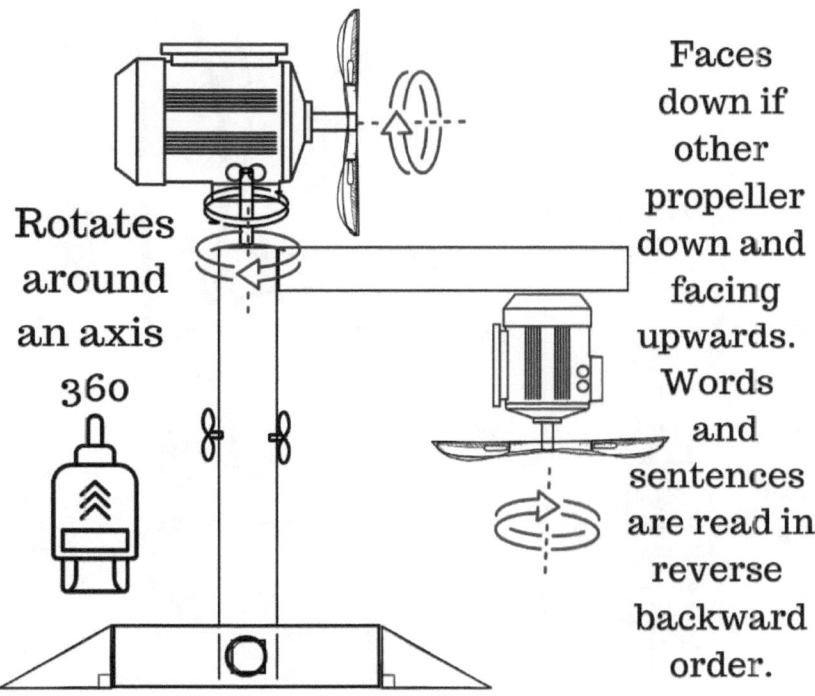

Rotates around an axis 360

Faces down if other propeller down and facing upwards. Words and sentences are read in reverse backward order.

Propeller now facing inwards

Rotates around
an axis 360

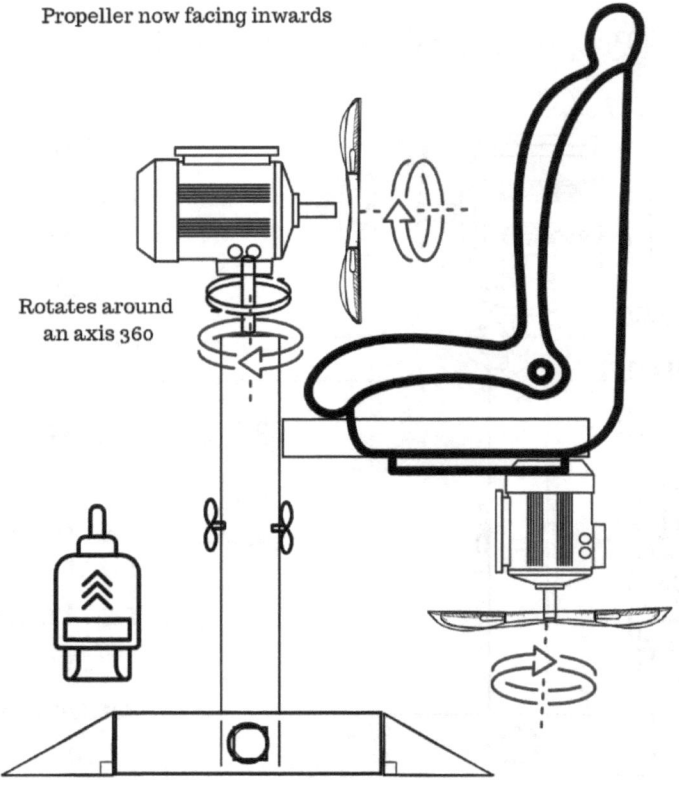

Invention 1a The Car Seat

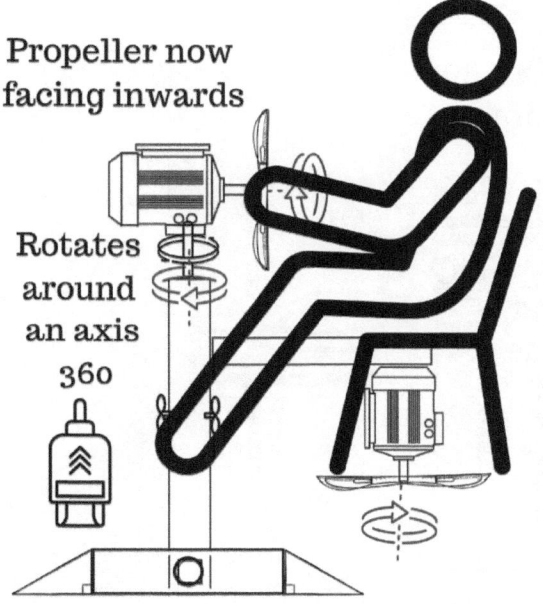

Propeller now
facing inwards

Rotates
around
an axis
360

Invention 1a The Car Seat

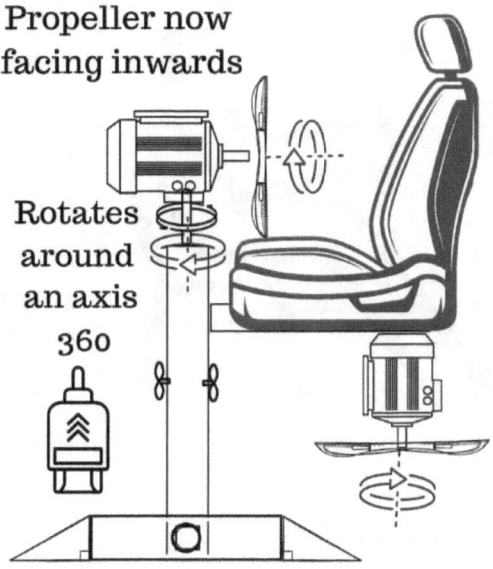

Propeller now
facing inwards

Rotates
around
an axis

360

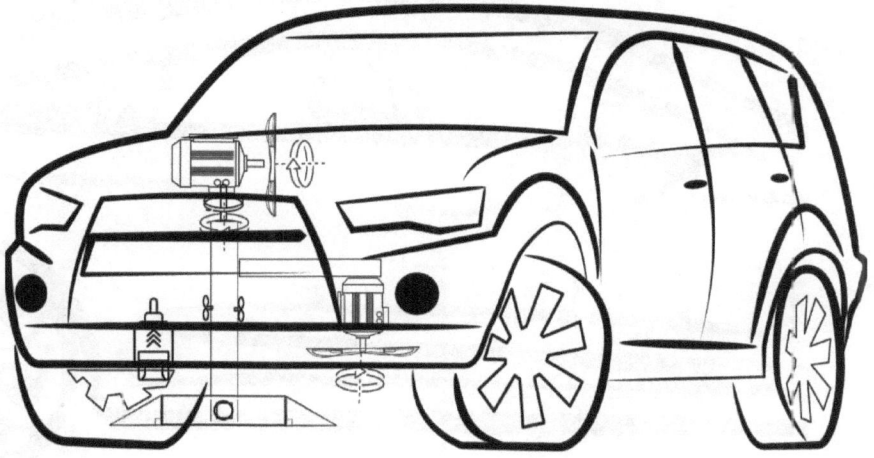

Invention 1a The Car Seat

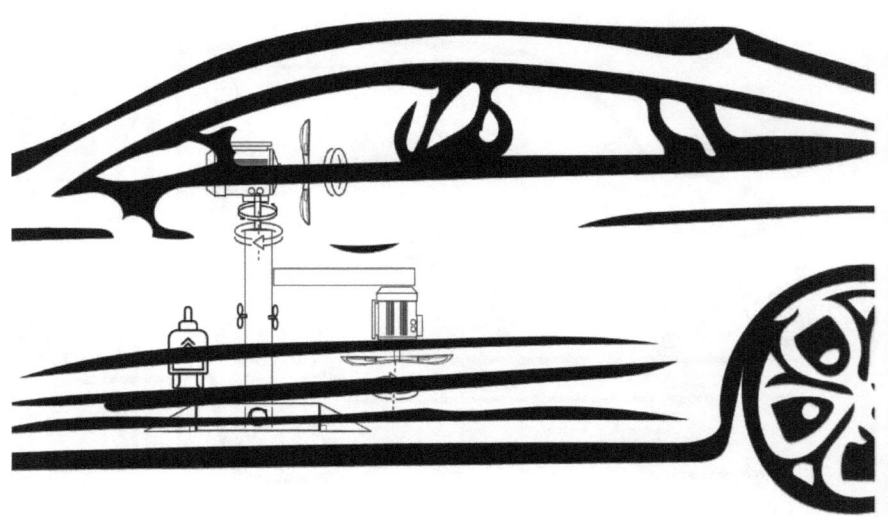

Propeller now facing inwards

Rotates around
an axis 360

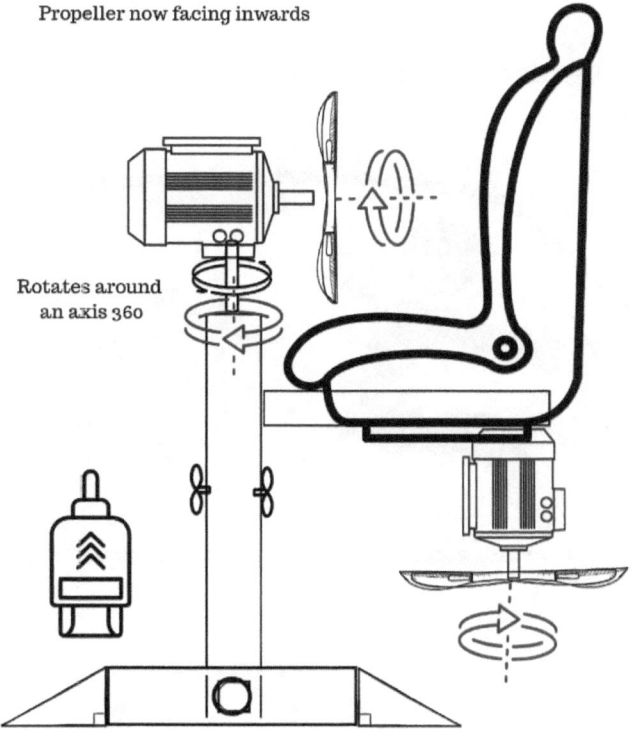

Invention 1a The Car Seat

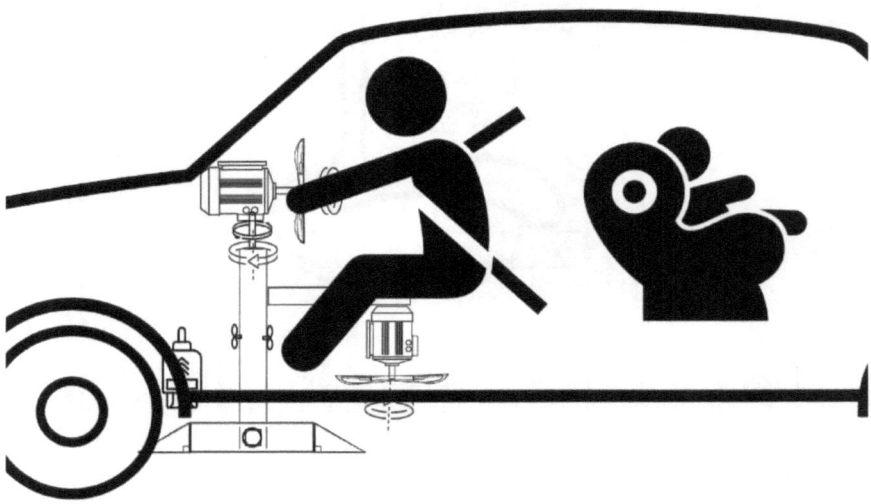

Effects of pushing brain thoughts out of the brain when mouth is closed, and frontal rotary propeller is switched off.

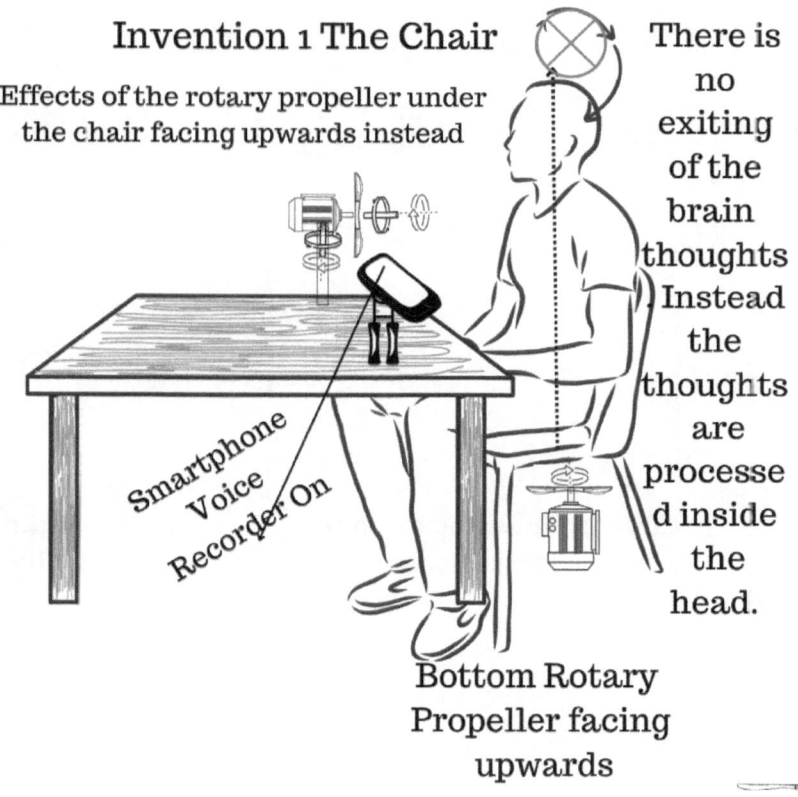

Invention 1 The Chair

Effects of the rotary propeller under the chair facing upwards instead

There is no exiting of the brain thoughts Instead the thoughts are processed inside the head.

Smartphone Voice Recorder On

Bottom Rotary Propeller facing upwards

Invention 1 The Chair

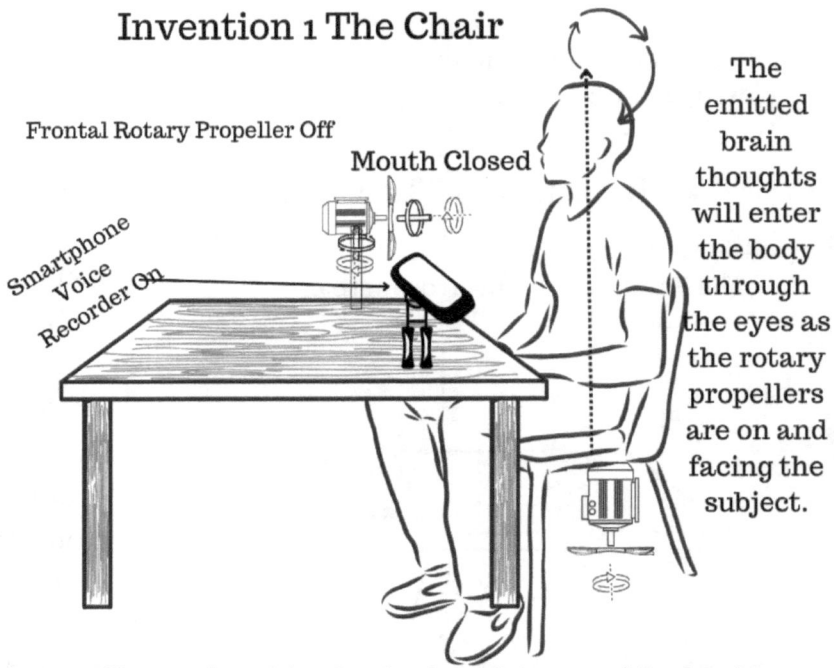

Frontal Rotary Propeller Off

Mouth Closed

Smartphone Voice Recorder On

The emitted brain thoughts will enter the body through the eyes as the rotary propellers are on and facing the subject.

Effects of pushing brain thoughts out of the brain when mouth is closed and frontal rotary propeller is switch off.

Invention 1 The Chair

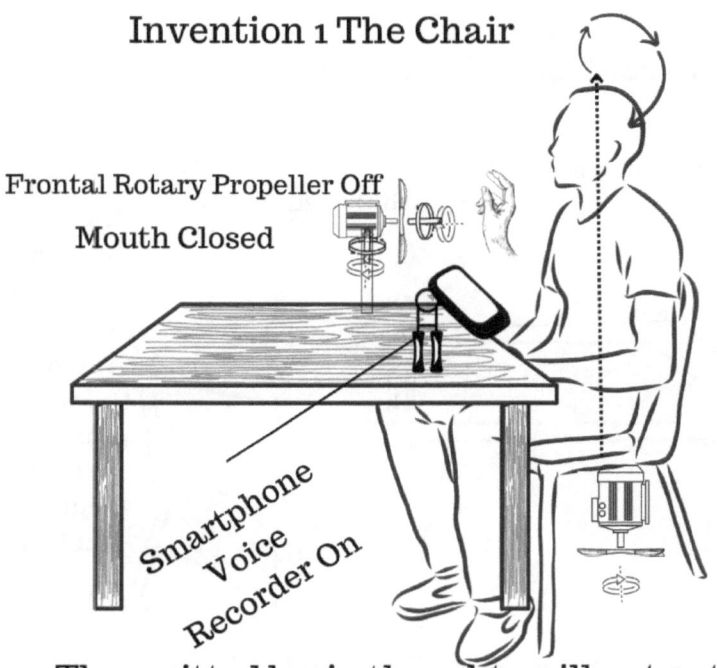

Frontal Rotary Propeller Off

Mouth Closed

Smartphone Voice Recorder On

The emitted brain thoughts will not enter the brain on the left side of the brain. No entry and the flow of the magnetic field is disjointed not complete

Invention 1 The Chair

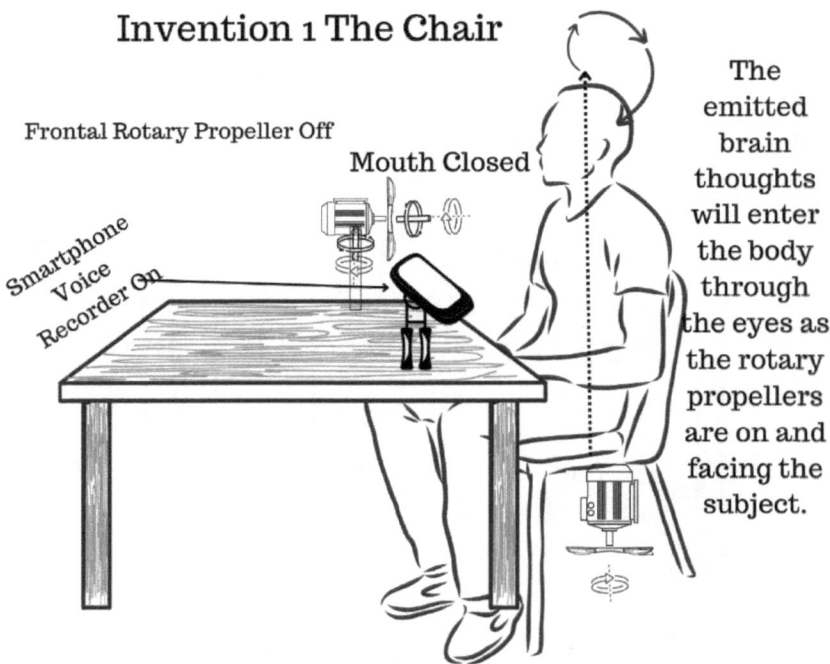

Frontal Rotary Propeller Off

Mouth Closed

Smartphone Voice Recorder On

The emitted brain thoughts will enter the body through the eyes as the rotary propellers are on and facing the subject.

Effects of pushing brain thoughts out of the brain when mouth is closed and frontal rotary propeller is switch off.

Invention 1 The Chair

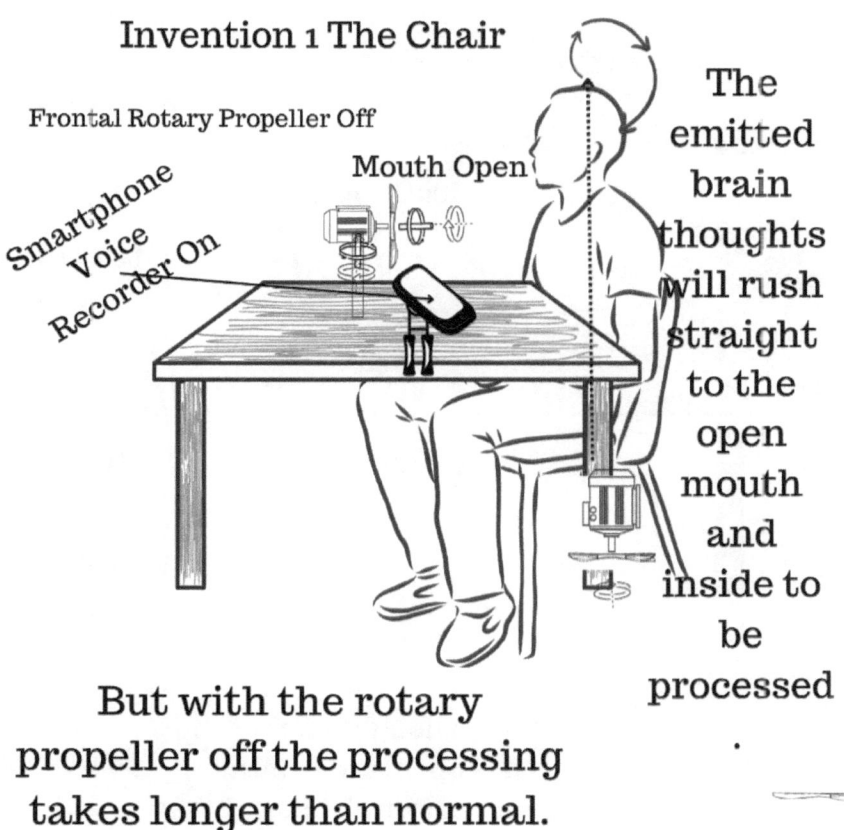

Frontal Rotary Propeller Off

Mouth Open

Smartphone Voice Recorder On

The emitted brain thoughts will rush straight to the open mouth and inside to be processed

But with the rotary propeller off the processing takes longer than normal.

Invention 1 The Chair

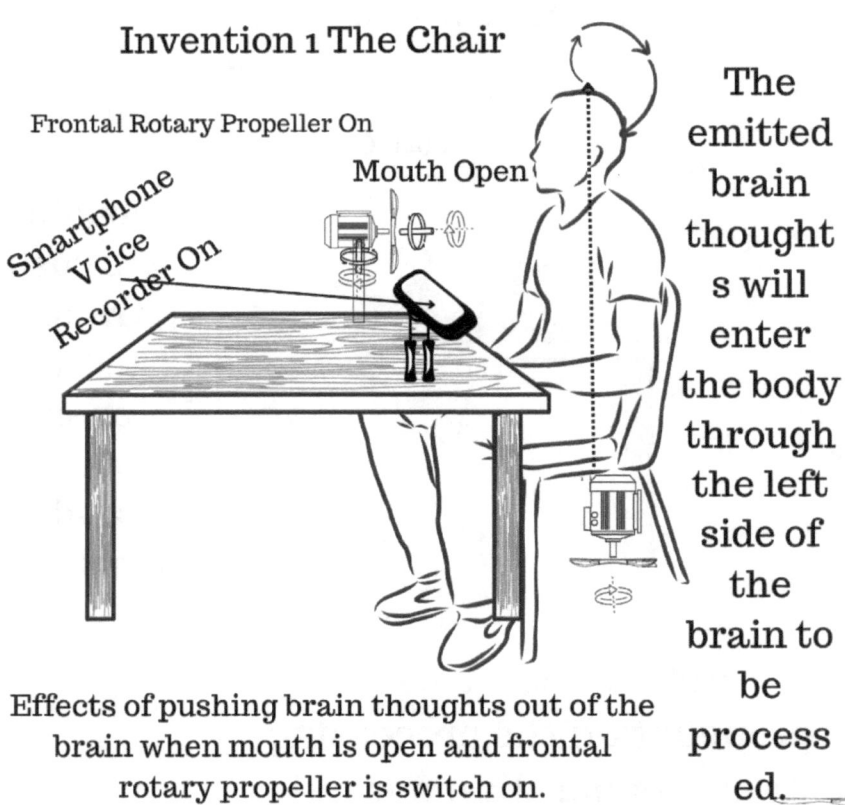

Frontal Rotary Propeller On

Mouth Open

Smartphone Voice Recorder On

The emitted brain thoughts will enter the body through the left side of the brain to be processed.

Effects of pushing brain thoughts out of the brain when mouth is open and frontal rotary propeller is switch on.

Invention 1 The Chair

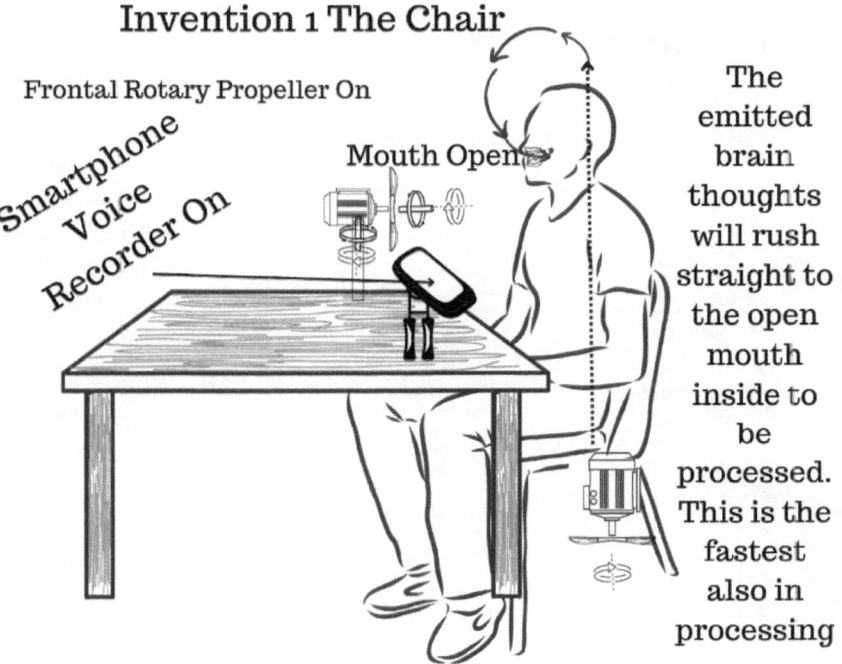

Frontal Rotary Propeller On

Smartphone Voice Recorder On

Mouth Open

The emitted brain thoughts will rush straight to the open mouth inside to be processed. This is the fastest also in processing.

Effects of pushing brain thoughts out of the brain when mouth is open and frontal rotary propeller is switch on.

Invention 1 The Chair

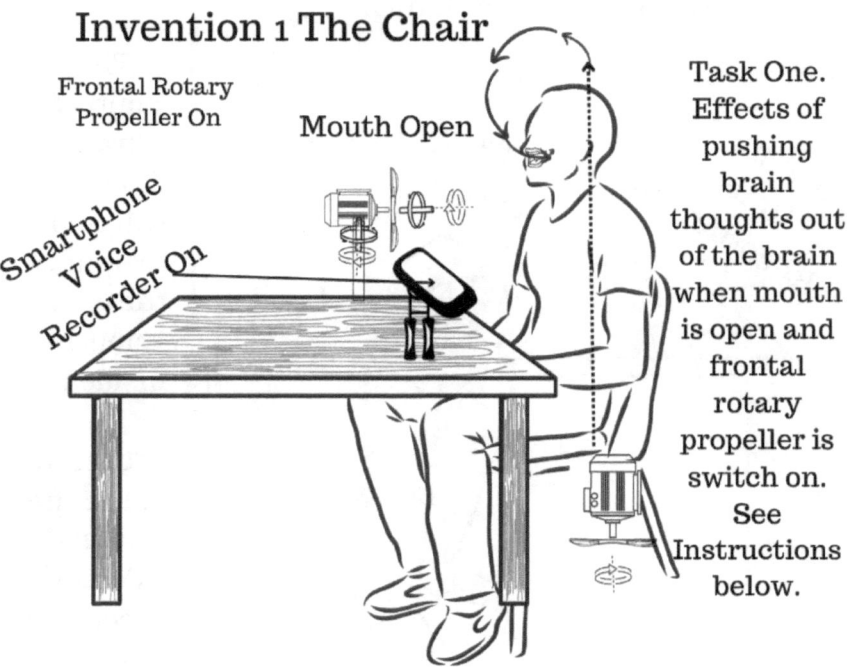

Frontal Rotary Propeller On

Mouth Open

Smartphone Voice Recorder On

Task One. Effects of pushing brain thoughts out of the brain when mouth is open and frontal rotary propeller is switch on. See Instructions below.

The emitted brain thoughts will rush straight to the open mouth inside to be processed.
This is the fastest also in processing.

Task One.
Effects of pushing brain thoughts out of the brain when mouth is open and frontal rotary propeller is switch on.
See Instructions below.

Task One.

Sit on a chair with the Oxy Cool Mini fan facing down and connected.
Connect frontal rotary propeller as above and switch it on. Switch smartphone in front of you to voice recorder. Put finger on the start recording button but don't start until next task is done.

Smartphone with voice recorder on

Rotary propeller facing the subject

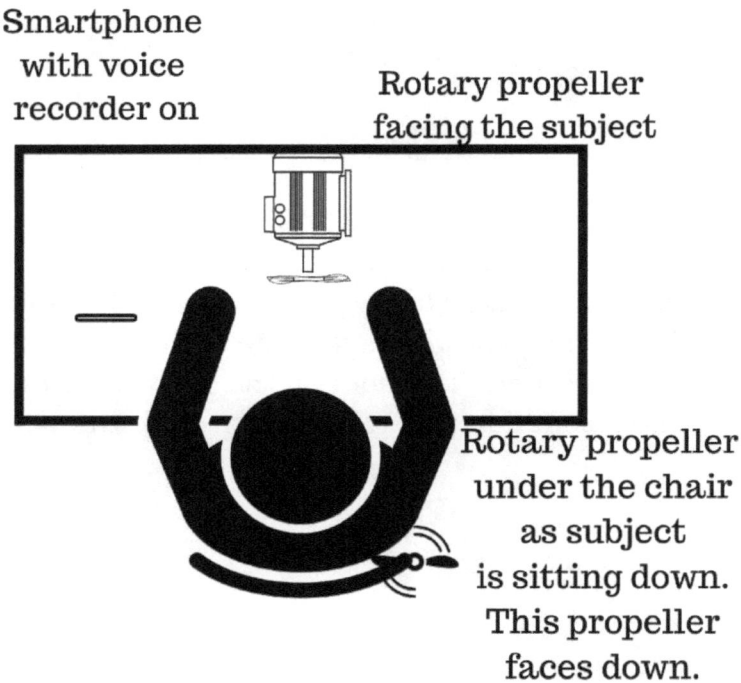

Rotary propeller under the chair as subject is sitting down. This propeller faces down.

Task One. Continues...

Sit straight making sure that the underneath rotary propeller is pointing to right buttock that sits deep into the chair.

Press the start recording button on smartphone's voice recorder.

Think about a word that has both a name and action as definitions. Take sex for example. It can refer to difference between male and female. Or an act as making love. Or simply a reference to sex organs.

Think about the word sex. If you have connected everything perfectly. Then if you listen very carefully you can feel the magnetic field created by the rotary propeller underneath the seat pushing the generated thoughts up. It only happens just after thinking of something.

Task One. Continues...

Listen very carefully for the exiting of the brain thoughts. After several times of practices, you will be able to tell when the thoughts have exited. It will be a pop like that of a champagne bottle opening sound.

Instantly open your mouth or just after you think of the word or action. The rotary propeller will be rotating. The body will go through stages explained in volume one chapters one to four.

The last stage can be felt if the rotary propellers are on. You can hear silently as far away the letters being arranged and a sound being made first on the right side and then on the left side. Once the words are passed through the middle of the tongue then you can hear what your thoughts were.

Our software will enhance this process.

After about 45 seconds that is if you have thought about the word sex then stop the recordings or as soon as you have heard the revelations.

Like feedback of what you were thinking about.

The mirror image of the body makes it act as if it is talking to itself. It is designed to do everything in two but as mirror images. One reads the word normally and the other reads the same word as in reverse that is backward.

Our software relies on the fact that everything we experience, and think is stored in the brain in different locations and classified according to a specific system. When a person thinks about sex for example. The brain will look for all these locations. It will check for the sex whether male or female.

Then to sex as an act meaning it will send a search down your genitals and bundle these results assigning binary numbers and changing letters of the word being searched either adding double SS EE XX or removing depending on the stage.

Then after being read backward the next step will then read, it correctly.

It is like a snake that goes forward then turns to face where it came from but starts going where it was going but backward until it reaches a corner then at the corner turn to face the correct way it is going.

Stop the Oxy Cool smartphone fan rotary proper in front of you that is on the Viido selfie stick. Switch off or simply unplug the Oxy mini fan underneath the chair. Now open the files folder on the smartphone and look for the voice recorder. You will not have said anything loudly. We are recording brain thoughts that are silent. First, we need to amplify this to levels we can detect.

Even though if you play this voice recording you can't hear anything. The brain's thoughts will have been recorded. Search on google for "Increase an MP3 volume online."

Select:

OnlineConverter.com

https://www.onlineconverter.com › increase-mp3-volu...

This free tool can help you increase or decrease the volume of MP3 audio. If the volume of your MP3 music is very light, it can make the sound louder, ...

Upload the file and click Convert the download after its volume has been increased.

Keep this MP3.

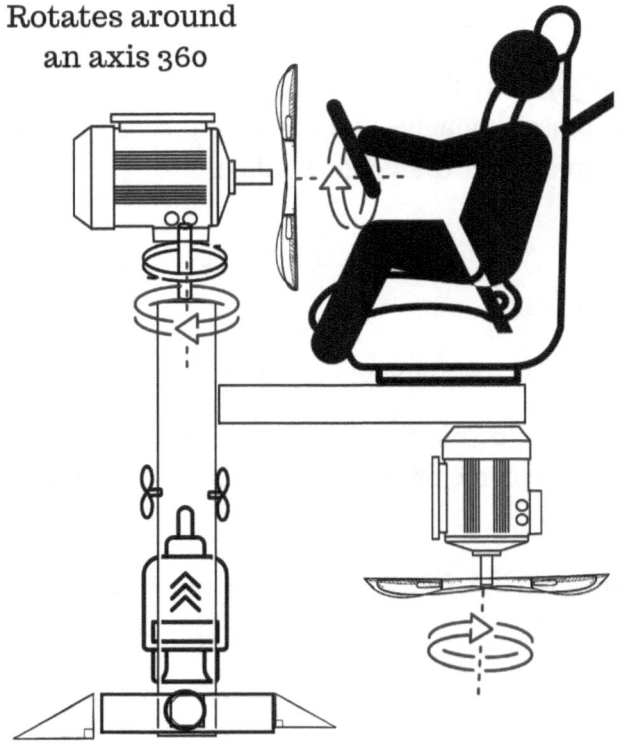

Rotates around an axis 360

Propeller now facing inwards.

Faces down if another propeller down and facing upwards. Words and sentences are read in reverse backward order.

This invention is also very suited to cars. The device can be incorporated as part of the car with the propeller being fitted facing downwards on the car driver seat. The rotary propeller in front can be fitted behind the steering wheel or as part of the steering wheel if it does not obstruct driving. All this can easily be incorporated into cars to guide drivers when driving. Their brain thoughts while driving can be fed into our software program to enable us to guide them. If they start losing concentration.

CHAPTER TWO

Grabbing Thoughts from the air.

Effects of pushing brain thoughts out of the brain when mouth is closed first then opened to eat the thoughts and frontal rotary propeller is switch off.

One can literally grab thoughts after they are emitted from the brain and open the mouth to eat the thoughts.
The body will go on to process these thoughts as if they have entered the body the normal way.

Invention 1 The Chair

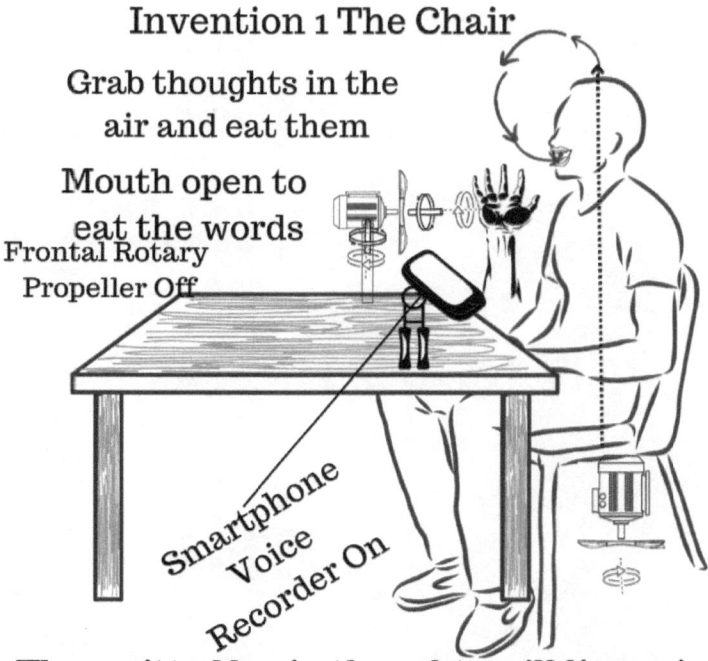

Grab thoughts in the air and eat them

Mouth open to eat the words

Frontal Rotary Propeller Off

Smartphone Voice Recorder On

The emitted brain thoughts will linger in the air first grab the thoughts in your hands and open your mouth then eat the thoughts to be processed.

Task Two.

Now that we have our Mp3 we must test it. We must set up the system so that we can check if the recording worked.

Items for task two.

1. Smartphone.
2. Two Oxy smartphone fans.
3. Juice power bank
4. Selfie stick with an already mounted juice bank and a smartphone fan.
5. A laptop at the workstation.

Detailed Specifications of The Brain Decoding Device. Volume II A Complete Step-by-Step Guide.

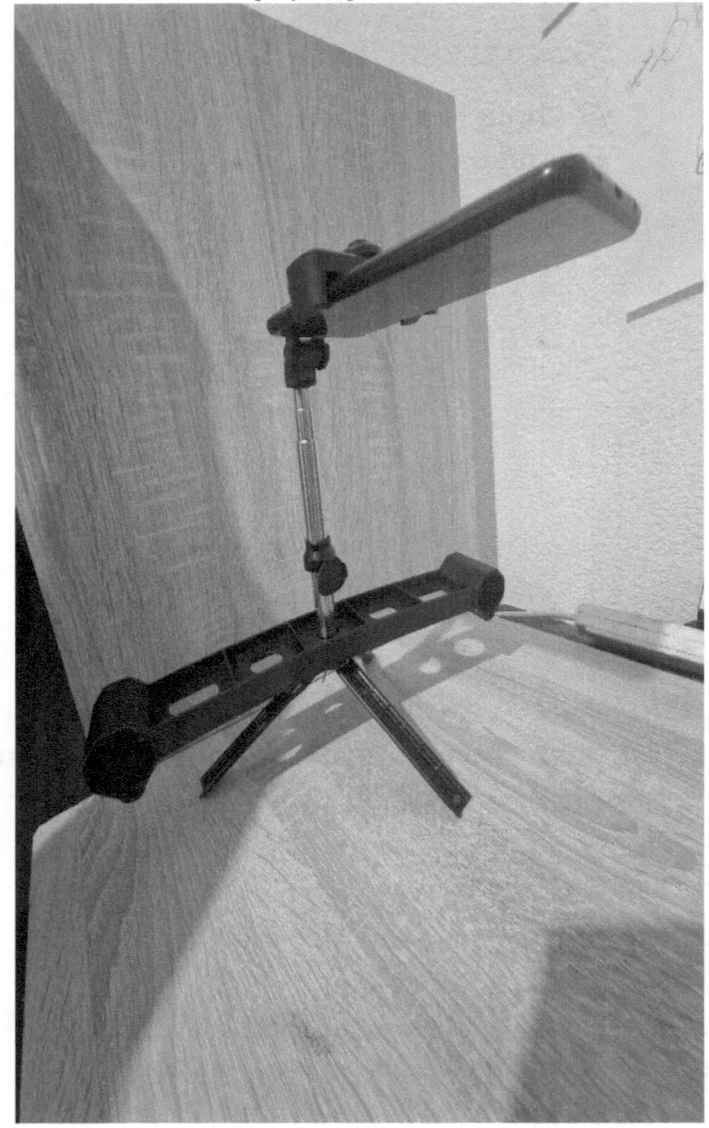

6. Connect the smartphone fan to the smartphone and place this on the left-hand side parallel to the raised screen of the laptop.
    Then connect the smartphone fan to the Juice power bank and place this on the left side.

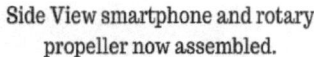

Side View smartphone and rotary
propeller now assembled.

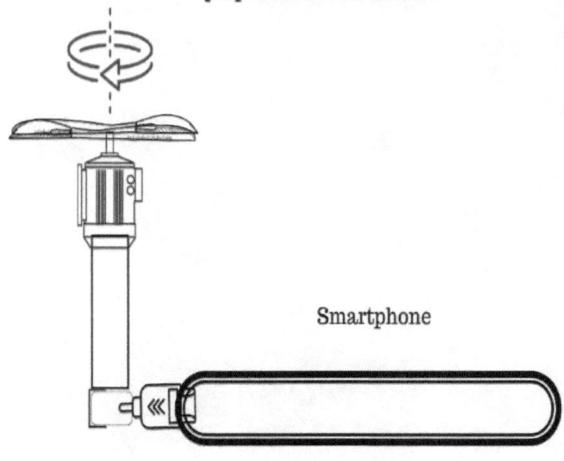

Smartphone

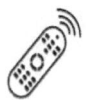

In advanced stages we will use the second smartphone for software interaction and advanced recordings and brain decoding.

Rotary Propeller 1

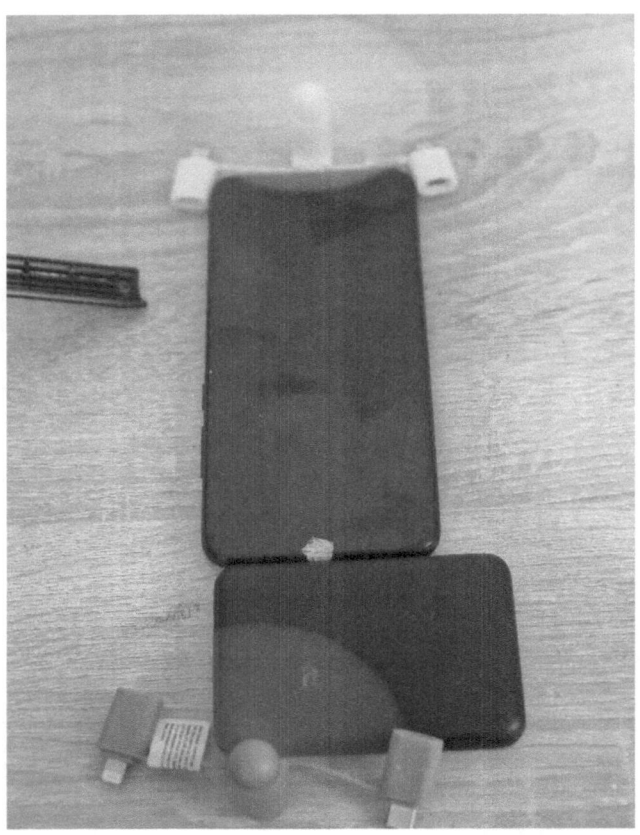

The side view of the op end rotary propeller and how it is connected to the brain decoding device.

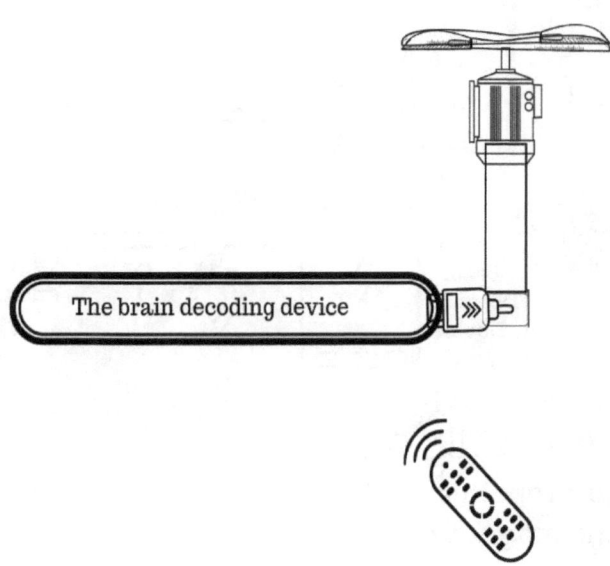

The Ultimate setting for the Brain Decoding Device. It works tried and tested.

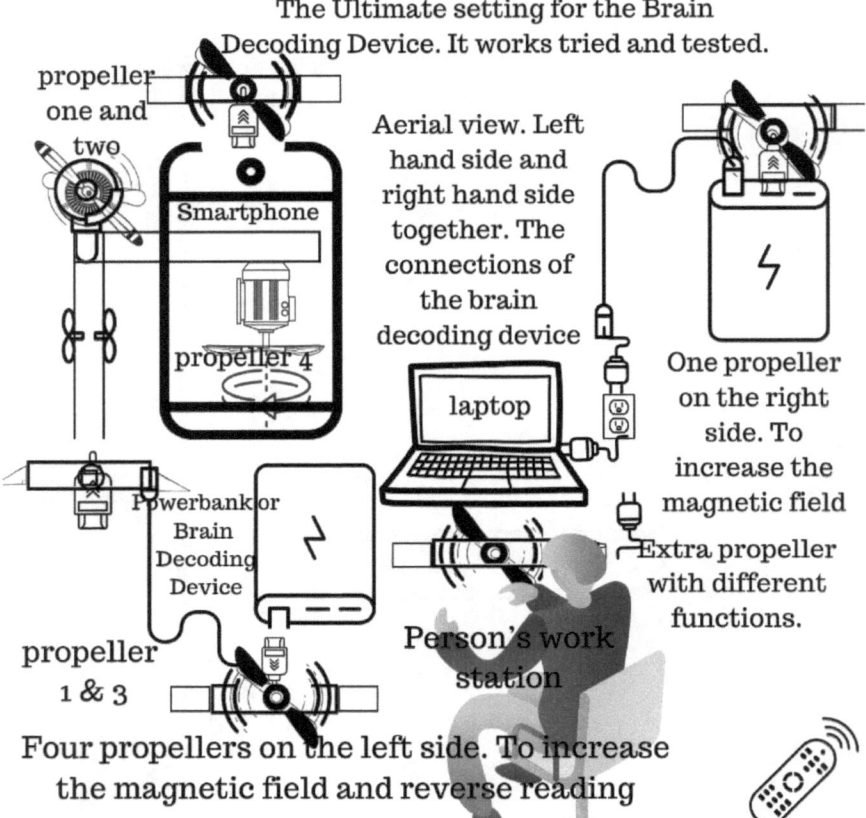

propeller one and two

Aerial view. Left hand side and right hand side together. The connections of the brain decoding device

Smartphone

propeller 4

laptop

One propeller on the right side. To increase the magnetic field

Powerbank or Brain Decoding Device

Extra propeller with different functions.

propeller 1 & 3

Person's work station

Four propellers on the left side. To increase the magnetic field and reverse reading

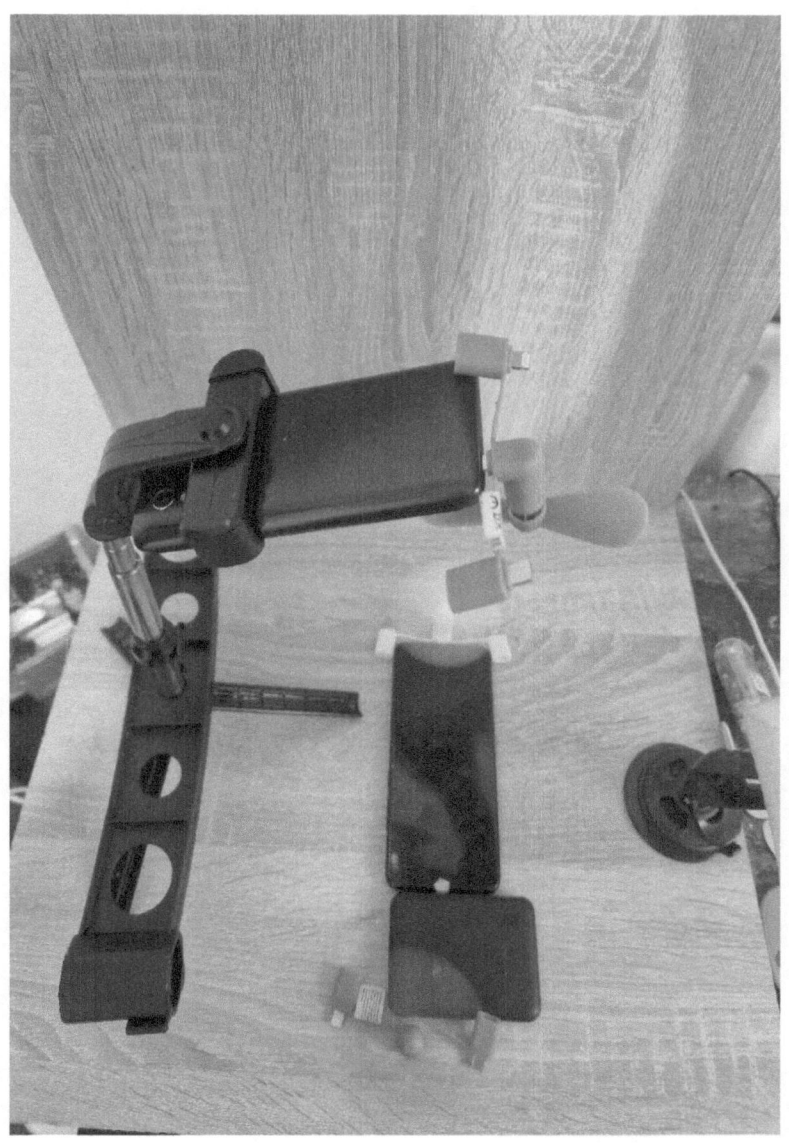

Currently the Juice Power-bank has replaced the brain decoding device in the image above. We will advance with time.

Below is the left side of the brain decoding device setup.

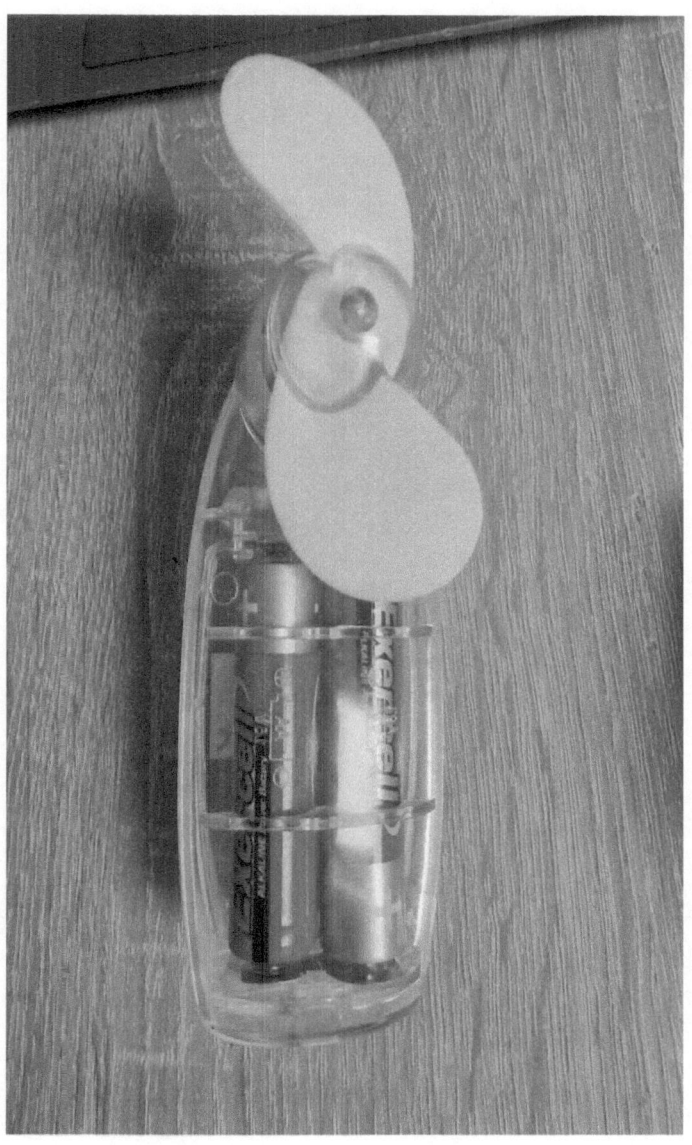

Now we will need a different kind of propeller.

We want one that is lower to the ground that points at the center of
the laptop.

This is model number SUM-3616 which costs only $2 from a
pound shop. This is the side view of the magnet. It is battery-
powered with two AA batteries.

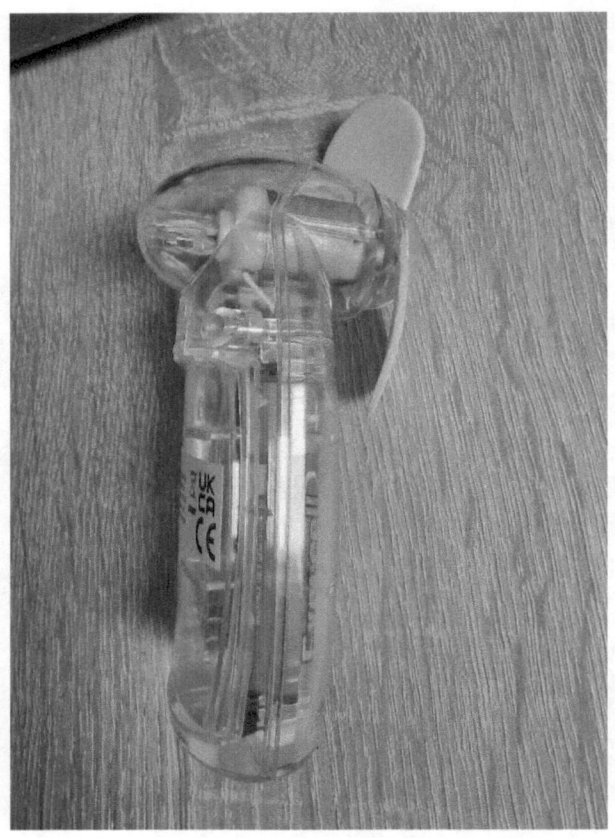

We want to replay our recording when we thought about the word sex and recorded that.
Get that MP3 that we increased volume.
Transfer to the laptop or computer. It is better on a computer or Laptop than on a phone. Nevertheless, a phone can do the job if you have an extra smartphone.

Open the MP3 using an MP3 player. Play it.
This should be the left side of the laptop on the workstation.
This should be the center of the laptop with that extra propeller close to the screen anywhere between 20 to 20 cm. This rotary propeller should be facing the laptop screen as here.
It should be in the middle of the screen ideally and rotating.
Now play that MP3 and listen to it.
You will not hear words or sounds the normal way, but the MP3 and the magnetic effect will make you say the thoughts with your mouth and your lips.

You will say the word you were thinking of yourself aloud. Your mouth will move by itself.
If that does not work, then you need to check if your setting is correct first.
Visit www.twofuture.world

Or click here.
https://twofuture.world/brain-commands

You must scroll down until you reach the Brain Commands Speaking. The page should be like the below image.

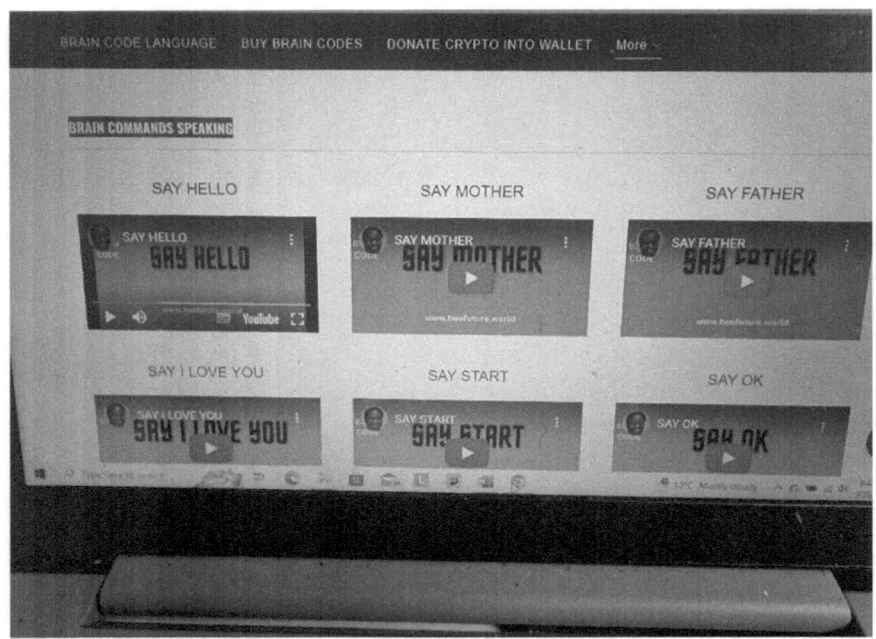

Play all one-by-one repeating to make sure that you can "hear" the words being said.
The left side must only have the following.

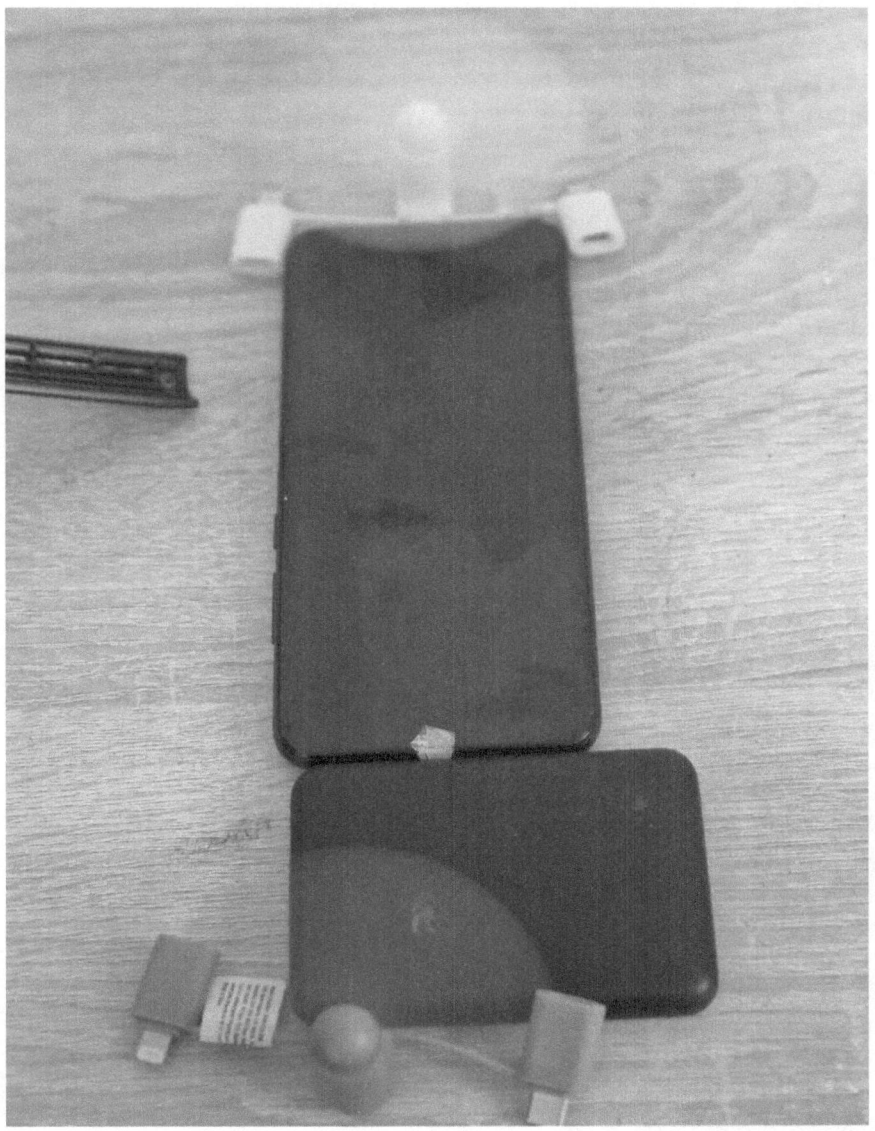

Only two rotary propellers were working and connected.

The rotating propeller must be at the center of the laptop.
You must be able to speak the words.

Now repeat the task and choose another word. Any word. Then after converting the recorded MP3 by increasing the volume. Now test it again. Replay while the third rotary propeller is at the desk just in front facing the laptop or computer screen.

Replay the thoughts in reverse. That is from backward first to the front.

The setting for replay in reverse is slightly different.

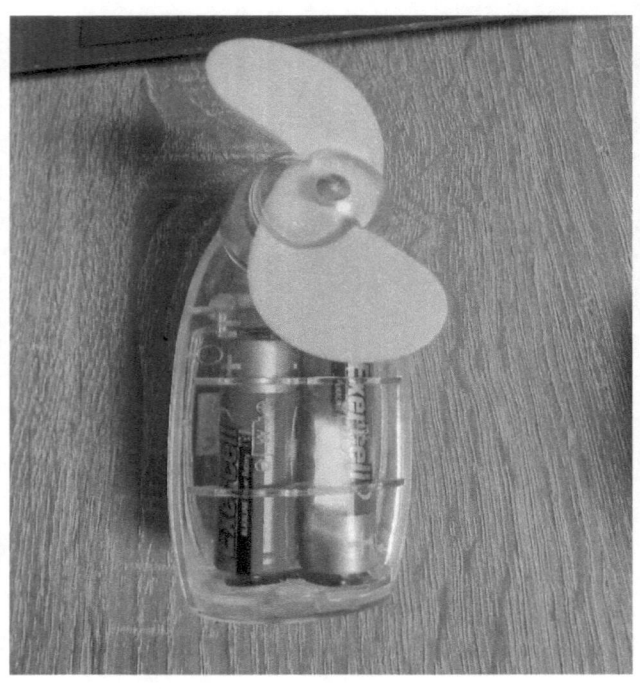

Repeat the below setting.

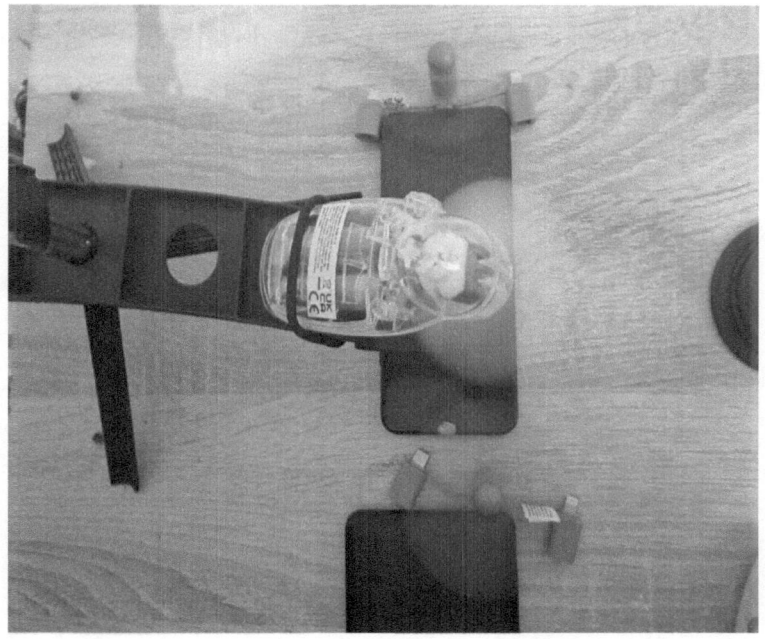

Now get the handheld propeller.

1. Switch it on and turn it upside down so that it points down to the above settings. Place it in the middle of the two rotary propellers and 22cm above the ground.

In the above photo, we used an already made hanging rotating bridge that can be rotated at a right-angle to the left-hand settings so that the handheld propeller can be suspended over this setting. If the propeller is rotating and if you play any recording or click here
https://twofuture.world/brain-commands

You must scroll down until you reach the Brain Commands Speaking. The page should be like the below image.
Now play all.

You will find out that.
Say Hello
 Will be replayed as Hello Say.
Say I love you will be replied as You love I say.
Say Mother will be replied as Mother Say.
Say Father will be replayed as Father Say.

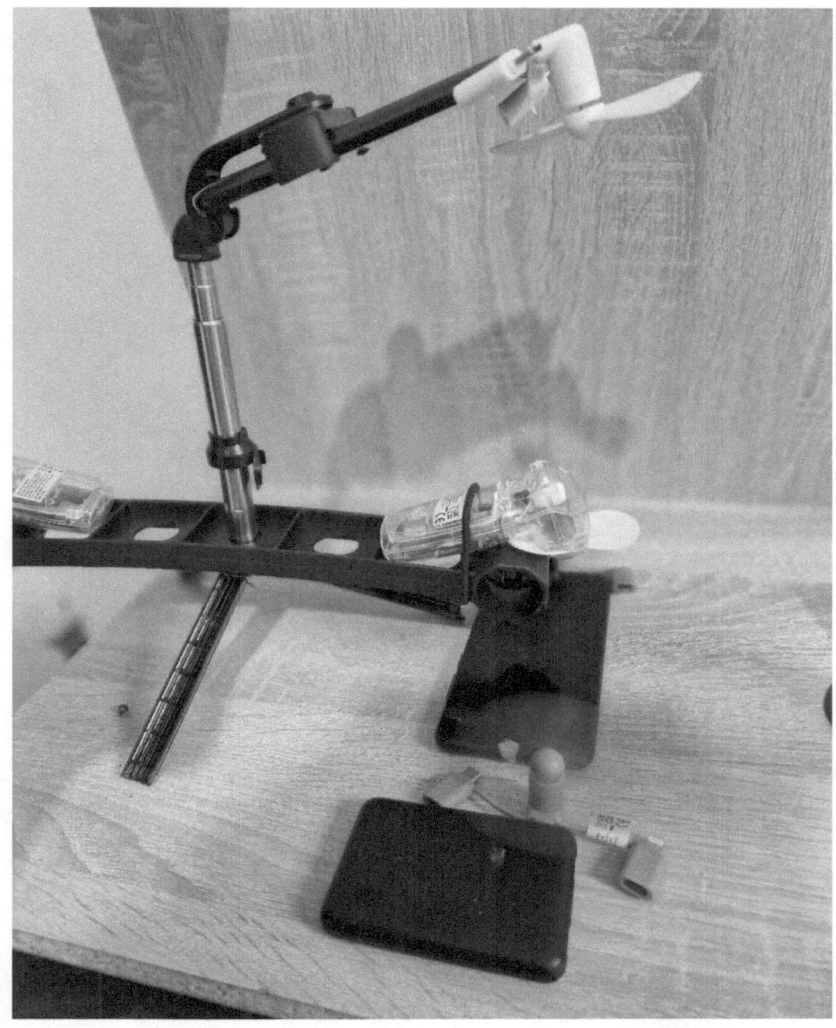

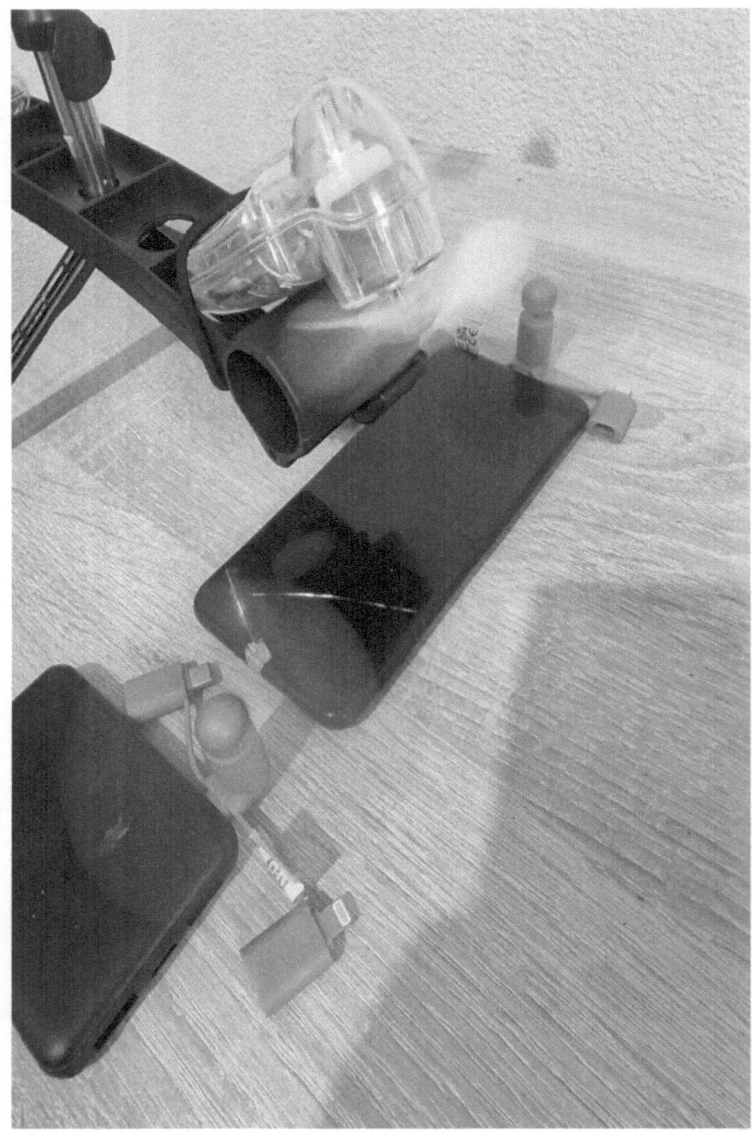

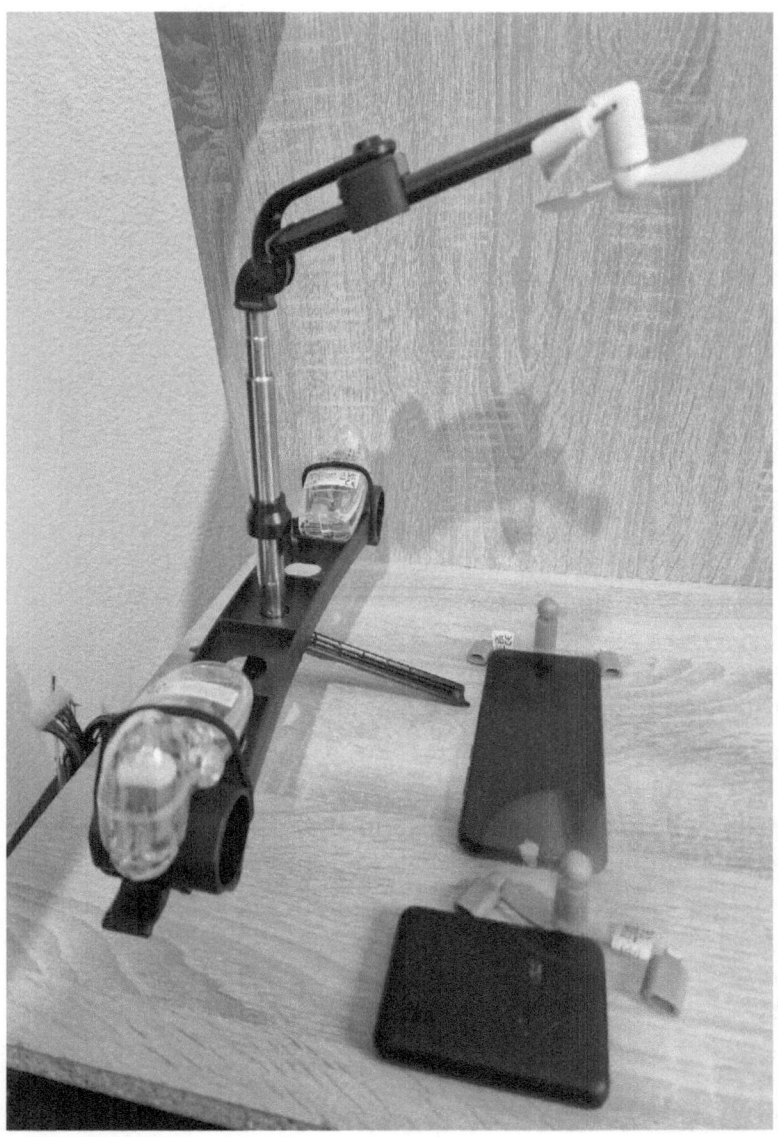

The above image has two possible perpendicular rotary function properties. The first one is the tall selfie stick with a mounted smartphone that is upside down. If a smartphone rotary propeller is connected and is also upside down this will provide the first reverse reading mode. If the height is above 40 cm the effect is reduced. The second lever-like bridge that can be rotated is mounted above so that it is at least above 22 cm. At any height below this, the reverse effect will not take place. It takes place best at 22 cm above the level where the left side setting is.

Now look at the above situation where we have two propellers at right angles to the left side settings. If we connect both rotary propellers perpendicular to the left side settings below this is the effect, we get.
The repetition Effect.
Two rotary propellers, one above the other, have the effect of causing the words to be repeated.

Say Hello will now become Say Hello Hello Hello Hello Hello.
Say Mother will now be replayed as Say Mother Mother Mother Mother.
Say I love you will now be replayed as Say I love you love you love you.
Say Father will now be replayed as Say Father Father Father Father Father.

Effect of rotating the propeller that is switched on the far side but still at a right angle to the left side settings. As in the photo below.

If the far end perpendicular propeller is switched on, then this has the effect of repeating the first word.
Say Hello will now become Say Say Say Say Say Say Hello.
Say Mother will now be replayed as Say Say Say Say Say Mother.

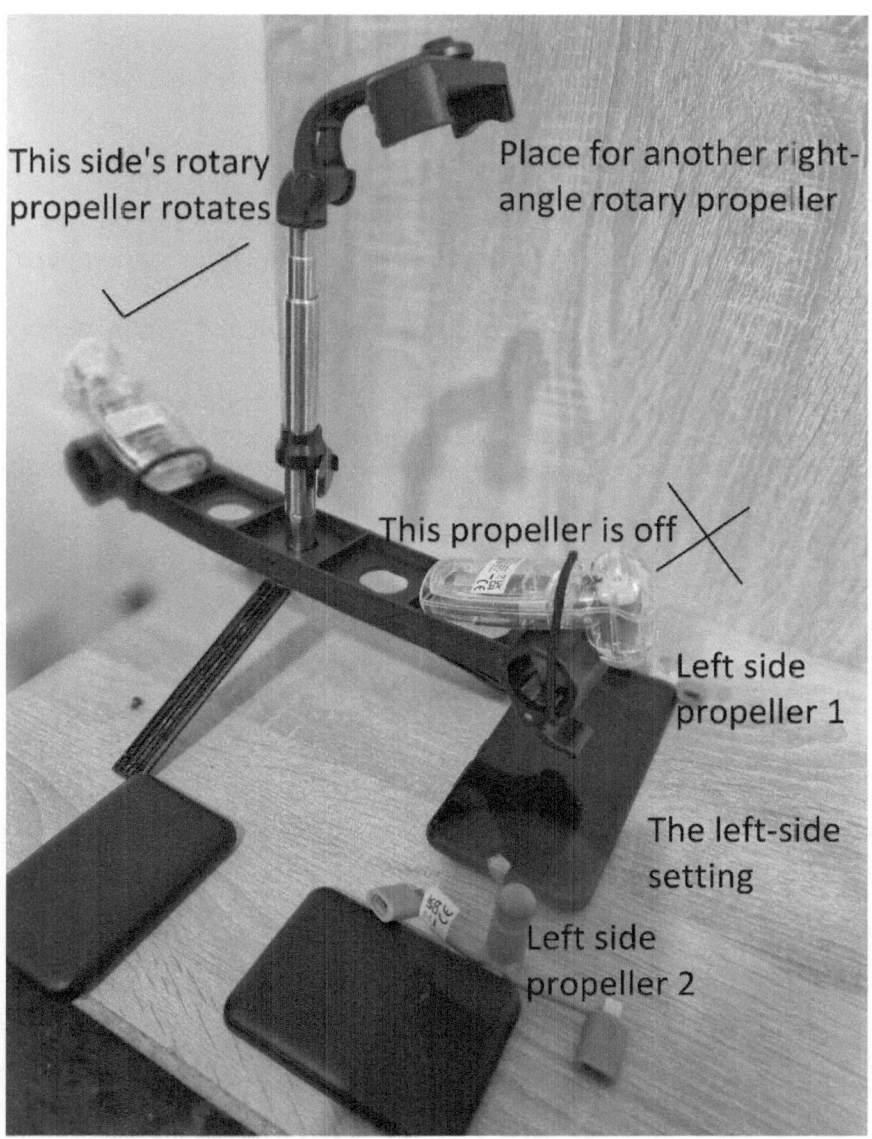

When testing the recorded MP3, you must set up the system as follows.

The left side must have everything we talked about. The middle part will have a laptop and another handheld propeller or one than can be placed on the surface but pointing at the laptop or computer screen.

Place the propeller at the center of the screen and within 20 cm range of the screen.

This image is on the left side. The next is the center. The third will be the right side. The third image is the right-hand side.

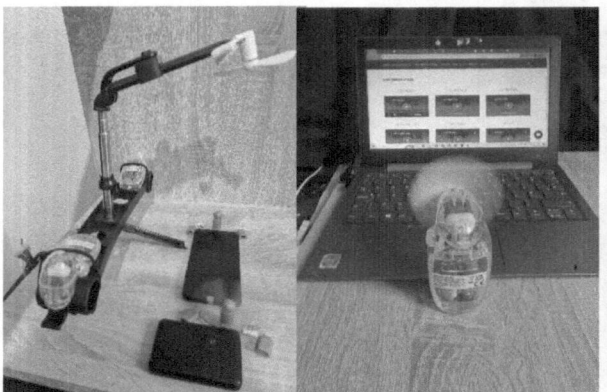 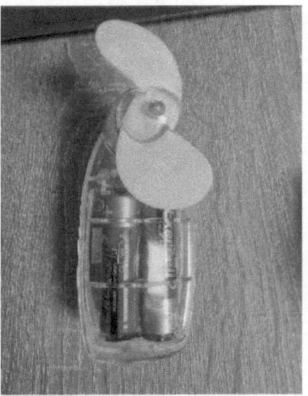

This is the booster side. Make sure you connected correctly, or this side can cancel out the flows of the electromagnetic flows.

I would advise setting up the left side and the center first only.

When this has worked, and you know what you are doing then add the third right side.

Note also that the third right side's propeller must face upward same as those on the left side [like a helicopter blade] not sideways.

CHAPTER THREE

Closing and opening of the entry and exit points on the brain by positioning of the rotary propellers.
Just as we open a port and push brain thoughts out of the brain into the atmosphere above the head, we can also use another rotary propeller position in such a way that it closes the port.

Note that we can simply switch off the propeller underneath the chair to stop thoughts from going out of the brain.

But we can also use another propeller to close the exit port.

A rotary propeller placed on top over the head of the subject facing down will have the effect of canceling the effect of the bottom under the chair propeller.

Effects of pushing brain thoughts out of the brain when there is another propeller added on top of the head

A suspended rotary propeller facing down or up on top of the one that is under the chair will cancel the exiting of brain thoughts

Invention 1 The Chair

A suspended rotary propeller facing down or
up on top of the one that is under the chair will cancel the exiting of brain thoughts

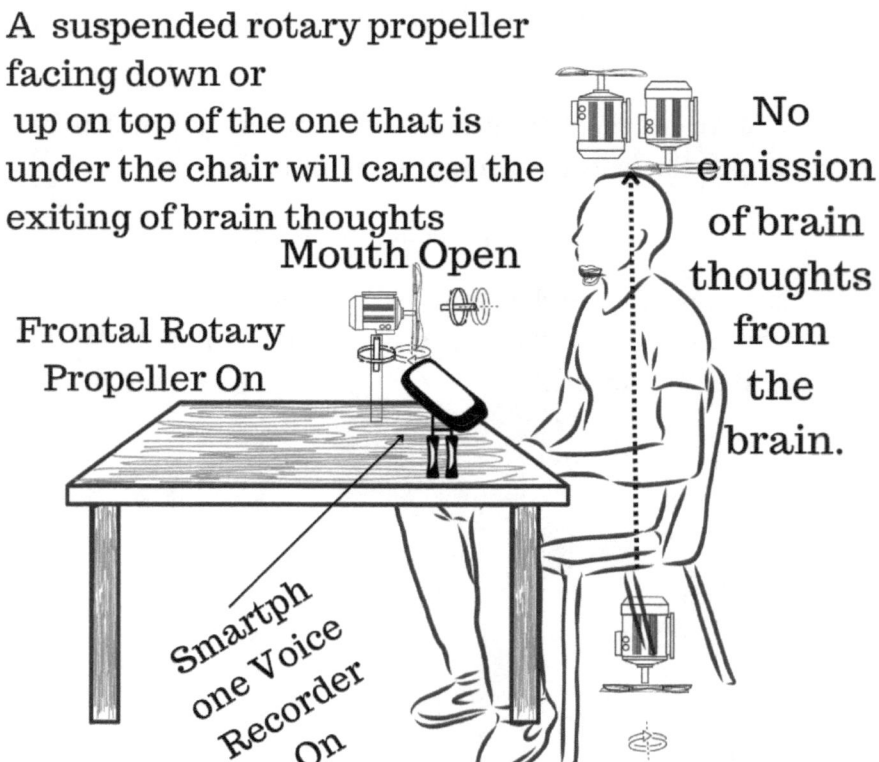

No emission of brain thoughts from the brain.

Mouth Open

Frontal Rotary Propeller On

Smartphone Voice Recorder On

What is the effect of adding another rotary propeller at the back of the front rotary propeller but facing the other side?

Effects of pushing brain thoughts out of the brain when mouth is open and frontal rotary propeller is switch on. Together with another added frontal propeller facing backward

Frontal Rotary Propeller On. Another propeller added facing the opposite.

The emitted brain thoughts will rush straight to the ears and is processed the same way but not as fast as through the mouth.
Try avoid the ear as entry point as it will tend to confuse the process later.

Invention 1 The Chair

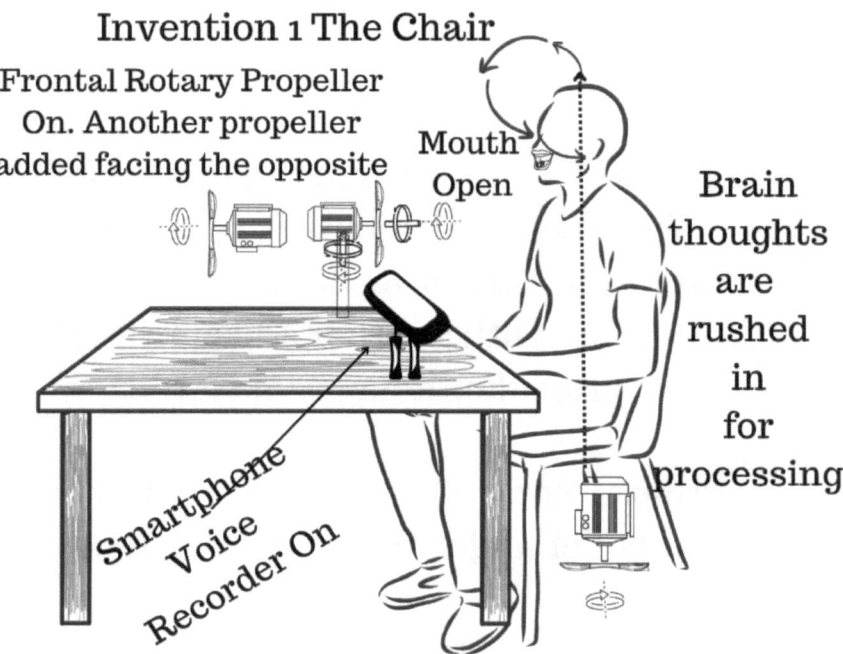

Frontal Rotary Propeller On. Another propeller added facing the opposite

Mouth Open

Brain thoughts are rushed in for processing

Smartphone Voice Recorder On

The emitted brain thoughts will rush straight to the ears and is processed the same way but not as fast as through the mouth.

CHAPTER FOUR

Invention 2 The Cloning /Duplicating and Doubling of the Brain Thoughts Device.

The main reason why we introduced rotary propellers in the first place is the need to know what a person is thinking at the same time or even before the person realizes what he or she was thinking about. We need a piece of the cake as well while the steel is still hot.

But how can we do this if it takes fractions of seconds for people to process their brain thoughts?

We must think fast and find a way to clone, duplicate, twin or double the person's thoughts so that we have a copy as well which we can decode.

The problem is the fact that we cannot deprive the person of his thoughts.

This is because it is possible to just intercept the person's thoughts and divert these thoughts to our brain decoder so that we know what the person was thinking about.

But lack of revelation and resolve.

If a person thinks about something, there must be a revelation when the thoughts are processed, and a person gets to know what he himself was thinking about. Secondly, this revelation gives answers to the person. When a person thinks he or she is asking the brain for any information regarding that thought.

Let us take for example a person who is thinking about a holiday in Egypt. That person is asking his brain what a holiday in Egypt is like. It is like asking if it has any information about him holidaying in Egypt. Or anything related to an Egyptian holiday past, now or futuristic.

So, the brain will search the brain about everything to do with Egypt. If we are to intercept and take the brain's thoughts without leaving anything for the brain to process. Then he will feel empty or hungry about the last thought. He was surely expecting answers but if this is not resolved the brain might not be able to process other thoughts properly.

In the end, he will know that something is wrong.

After all the process will be useless because even, he without this feedback will not know what he just thought about.

Therefore, we must find a way of providing a solution. One that will clone, twin, or duplicate the thoughts so that we have our copy we can use to decode the person's brain thoughts. That means not interfering with his or her system.

The Cloning Device.

Therefore, outright the purpose of a rotary propeller under the chair or car seat is to push a person's thoughts out so that we can make a copy of the thoughts so that we know what a person was thinking about.

Positioning of the cloning device.

Ideally, the cloning device must be close to the entry point after pushing the brain's thoughts out of the body.

But how do we get the thoughts into our cloning, duplicating, and twining devices?

There must be a diverter from the entry point to our cloning device. That also means there must be a reverse back to the entry point from our cloning device. This is because we must take the thoughts through our cloning device just to clone the thoughts so that we have our thoughts to work on.

Now we must send the diverted thoughts back to the brain to be processed. The ideal method is one that diverts from the entry point to the cloning device and diverts one back to the person's entry point.

We need a diverter.

Another rotary propeller smaller in size now on the left side of the chair can act as a diverter to the cloning device. In a car for example this is placed on the same driver's seat but close to the left side. The effect of this smaller rotary propeller is to divert entry from the entry point usually on the left side to where it is.

That means the cloning device must also be next to it. That is on the left side of the chair or car seat.

The Cloning Device.

The diverted thoughts are attracted to this position where a cloning device will be.

A cloning device since thoughts are like the air in the electromagnetic form they can be cloned if passed through a pipe or area that can pressurize these thoughts enough to split them into two with one diverted back for entry into the subject and the other sent to the decoder.

That means also that one of the chambers must have a needle diode or another rotary propeller that acts as the diverter as well. Therefore, another smaller rotary diverter back to the entry point.

This is the first option.

At the beginning of this book Volume II, I went further to explain what can be done to make thoughts be entered into the body at different points and situations. That means the thoughts do not necessarily have to enter the body through the entry point on the left side.

Thoughts can enter the body using any orifices on the body through the anus, vagina, ears, mouth, eyes, ears even though ears are not ideal.

The first option is through the mouth.

I explained earlier that the mouth is the fastest way. This is because everyone's body processes their thoughts according to each stage reached. Visit volume I to see all the stages of brain thoughts are processed. The mouth is as good as the final stages. This is because here saliva and the mouth network will assign a binary number once or twice just before the saliva dissolves these binary numbers making the alphabetical letters ready for the final processing in the jaws. Starting in the right law, then the left jaw then the middle of the tongue which is the part of the revelation.

The advantage is that this will offset the delay in diverting the brain's thoughts to our cloning device. Now the person can still receive the revelation at the same time as if the brain's thoughts were not diverted and delayed.

There are other ways. But I will look at these later in the book.

The effect of the other rotary propeller.

Once the thoughts are diverted to the left side of the same seat of the car driver or chair. After cloning the emitted brain thoughts will be stopped by the initial rotary propeller under the chair. The rotary propeller in the left side of the chair or car seat is also facing downward and this creates the trapping of the brain thoughts between the two propellers all under the seats. That makes the brain's thoughts travel to areas of low pressure, which are often the mouth or nose. If the mouth is open the thoughts are absorbed through the mouth. If closed, then enters the body through the nose or in worst cases through the eyes or even ears.

The Divertor
A rotary propeller on the left side of the same chair or seat of a car will act as divertor at the point of entry and a divertor to where it is.

The emitted brain thoughts will rush straight to the open mouth inside to be processed. This is the fastest also in processing.

First rotary propeller as the pusher out of the brain of thoughts

Second small rotary propeller as the diverter or attractor to itself. Meaning the cloning device must be near this diverter.

Invention 1 The Chair

The Divertor.

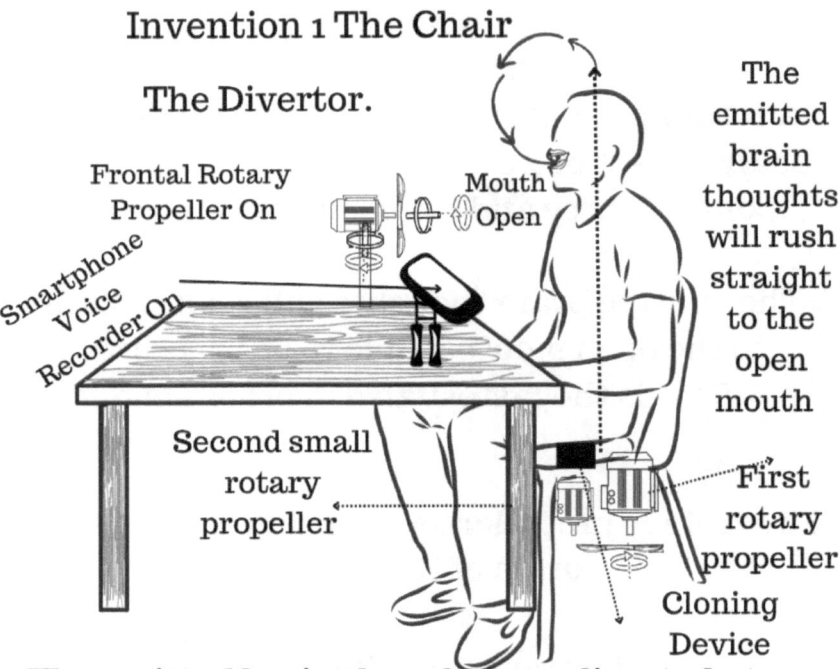

Frontal Rotary Propeller On

Mouth Open

Smartphone Voice Recorder On

The emitted brain thoughts will rush straight to the open mouth

Second small rotary propeller

First rotary propeller

Cloning Device

The emitted brain thoughts are diverted at the entry point to the place next or near the diverter to be cloned, twined and duplicated

Under driver's seat or chair

Two chambers to split and divert the thoughts

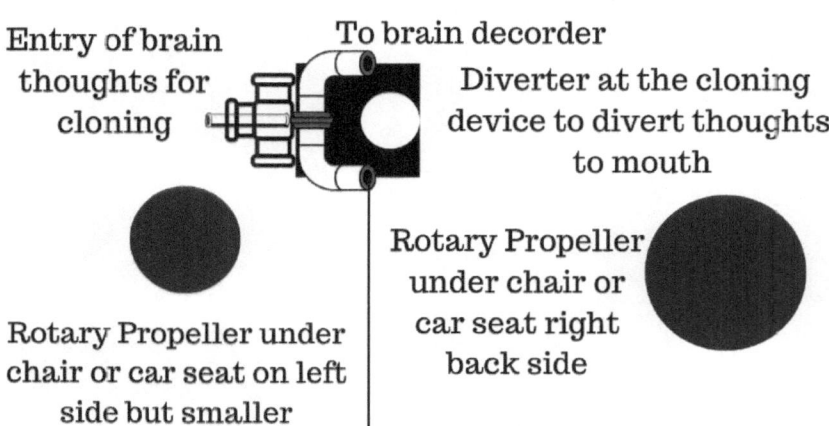

Entry of brain thoughts for cloning

To brain decorder

Diverter at the cloning device to divert thoughts to mouth

Rotary Propeller under chair or car seat right back side

Rotary Propeller under chair or car seat on left side but smaller

To mouth for absorption

Diverted to the mouth
Pressure from both side traps the cloned thoughts that in the end they travel to a low pressure in the mouth

We know what will happen to the absorbed thoughts entered through the mouth. Check-in volume one for explanations.
That means the diverted thoughts have been reentered but further down the processing stages. This will make up for the lost time done through diversion of the brain's thoughts.

The cloned thoughts are sent for decoding.

The thoughts that were cloned are sent as a copy of the original for processing. It goes through the same stages as illustrated in Volume 1.
After revelations, one can tell what a person was thinking about.

Detailed Specifications of The Brain Decoding Device. Volume II A Complete Step-by-Step Guide.

CHAPTER FIVE

Going Wireless.
Going forward we can make the device simple and to some extent replace it with Mac Bluetooth reference points.

Going forward the gadgets can be very miniature the size of an ear pad that can be fitted inside smartphones as part of all smartphones when we go global. The size will only reduce with time.

Reference points can be used just to denote where all these rotary propellers will be situated in space and time. The brain's thoughts will be diverted by a needle diode the size of a small button on a smartphone. The rotary propellers will be miniature but powerful. The seat can only have buttons with Bluetooth links where the entire system is in the bonnet of a car or inside a smartphone.

Rotary Propeller activated only when on demand.
Everything in this stage is done remotely and on-demand only. The propeller functions appeared but as virtual only represented by a Mac Bluetooth address. The action happens in the background and a virtual link is highlighted only.

Invention 1 The Chair
Everything happening in the background and only virtual points represented in the open air. The future.

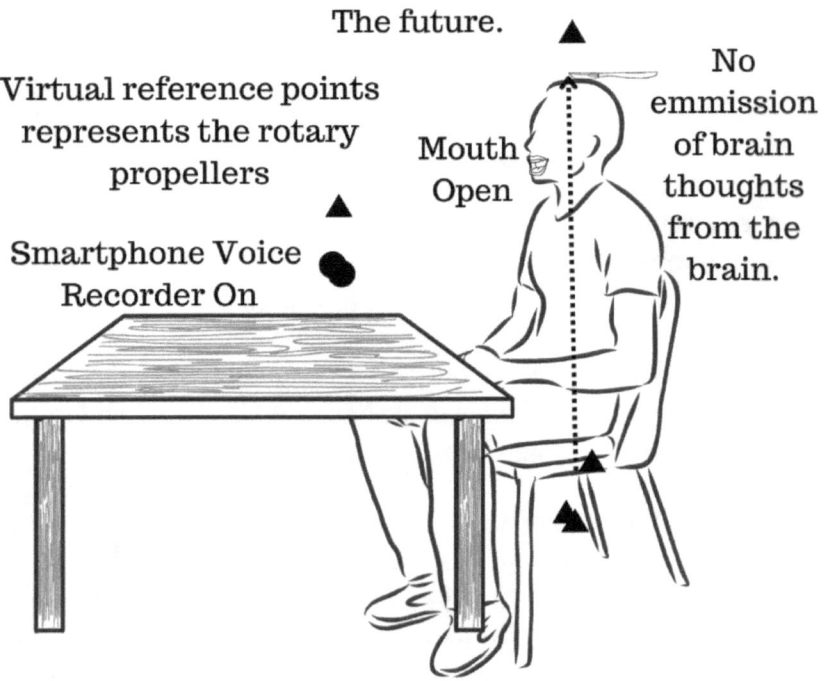

Virtual reference points represents the rotary propellers

Mouth Open

No emmission of brain thoughts from the brain.

Smartphone Voice Recorder On

Future Device as part of the Car Systems

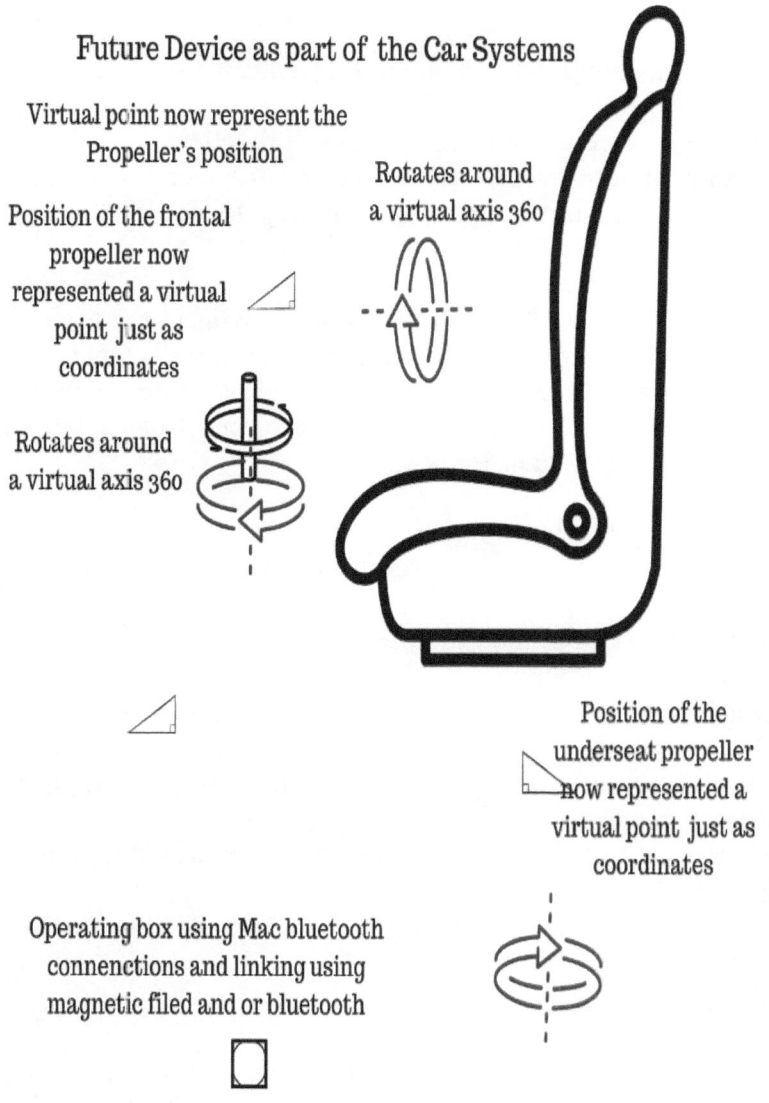

Virtual point now represent the
Propeller's position

Rotates around
a virtual axis 360

Position of the frontal
propeller now
represented a virtual
point just as
coordinates

Rotates around
a virtual axis 360

Position of the
underseat propeller
now represented a
virtual point just as
coordinates

Operating box using Mac bluetooth
connenctions and linking using
magnetic filed and or bluetooth

.... To be continued in Volume III........

Now while you are waiting for Volume III practice.

Now think about several words and record using the voice recorder. Process that is amplify and replay to see if this has worked.

Now record full thoughts not just words. Now use time to think of a subject and record for example for two minutes. Once you have stopped recording the thoughts using voice recorder. You can write down the thoughts word to word on a piece of paper before processing. Then check later for accuracy.

Then after that try this.

In one room set up as before. Ask someone to sit on the chair with a magnet at the bottom.

The person must close their mouth.

In another room.

You can buy another stronger rotary fan, the mini fan or bigger.

Now do the recording away from the person thinking.

Now we want to know what the other person was thinking in the lounge.

Use time to ask to start thinking for example at 8pm for two minutes.

A timer can be used.

Then in the study room synchronize the recording. At 8pm put a speaker in front of someone else but the speaker will be facing this other person who is recording. Record for two minutes.

Then do the conversion.

First to be sure ask the person thinking to first think also about his or her name. Then the thoughts.

The reason being that you will record thoughts that will also include others.

When checking later you can use the name as well to verify.

Now ask someone to sit in the chair and think f something and record at the same time.

Then you go and sit there and replay the recording at that same place and see if you can know the person's thoughts. The idea being that we can synchronize two events as if they are happening at the same time.

We must delay one event so that it matches the other.

Now ask someone to sleep and dream sitting there or set up a new station, use the propeller under the bed and record them while sleeping then process the recording and replay it and see if you know exactly what they have dreamed about.

The future is exciting stay tuned...

Volume III is coming soon.

Read all our other books.

Here is the complete series link.

https://play.google.com/store/books/series?id=a4MvGwAAAB BFmM

DAVID GOMADZA

I am the First Global President of The World.
I am going to introduce a new system of global governance and
planning. A new system that is spearheaded by advancement in
technology.
Technology shall be the driver of the economy and not wars as in
today's situation.

Detailed Specifications of The Brain Decoding Device. Volume II A Complete
Step-by-Step Guide.